NVQs IN NURSING
AND RESIDENTIAL HOMES

Other books of interest

Nursing in Nursing Homes
Linda Nazarko

Knowledge to Care
A Handbook for Care Assistants
Edited by
Christine McMahon
and
Joan Harding

Care of the Older Person
A Handbook for Care Assistants
Edited by
Christine McMahon
and
Ron Isaacs

Ethics and Values for Care Workers
Vic Tadd

Clinical Nursing Practice
in the Community
Edited by
M. Kenrick
and
K. Luker

Community Health Care Nursing
Edited by
D. Sines

NVQs IN NURSING AND RESIDENTIAL HOMES

Linda Nazarko
BSc (Hons) Gerontology, RN

Blackwell
Science

DISTRIBUTORS

Marston Book Services Ltd
PO Box 269
Abingdon
Oxon OX14 4YN
(*Orders:* Tel: 01235 465500
     Fax: 01235 465555)

North America
 Blackwell Science, Inc.
 Commerce Place
 350 Main Street
 Malden, MA 02148 5018
 (*Orders:* Tel: 800 759 6102
        617 388 8250
     Fax: 617 388 8255)

Canada
 Copp Clark Professional
 200 Adelaide Street, West, 3rd Floor
 Toronto, Ontario M5H 1W7
 (*Orders:* Tel: 416 597-1616
        800 815-9417
     Fax: 416 597-1617)

Australia
 Blackwell Science Pty Ltd
 54 University Street,
 Carlton, Victoria 3053
 (*Orders:* Tel: 03 9347-0300
     Fax: 03 9347-5001)

A catalogue record for this book is
available from the British Library

ISBN 0–632–04018–1

Dedication

With love to my husband whose enthusiasm
and encouragement helped turn a fireside chat into a book.

Thanks Ed

Contents

Preface

This is an exciting time for care assistants working in nursing and residential homes. In recent years the numbers of older people cared for in homes has risen enormously and more than a million older people are now cared for in homes. The growth in the numbers of old people in the population, changes in the health service, and the introduction of the Community Care Act have meant that people living in homes require higher levels of care than ever before. Since the mid-1980s homes have changed beyond all recognition. Standards have risen; now most homes offer single or double rooms which are carpeted and furnished to higher standards than before. Facilities which were once viewed as luxuries are now becoming standard. Older people, their families, social services departments and health authorities now expect higher standards of care from staff. At the same time the people cared for in homes require more help with the activities of daily living than ever before.

The role of care assistants has changed dramatically. Many experienced care assistants have undertaken training within the home, attended study days and spent time visiting clinics and observing specialists at work. Until recently these achievements were not always recognized. The introduction of National Vocational Qualifications (NVQs) enables care assistants, for the first time, to gain a qualification which demonstrates to employers their level of skills.

Care assistants studying for NVQ qualifications work through a closely monitored programme which increases their level of knowledge and enables them to gain credit for practical skills. NVQ qualifications enable care assistants to increase this knowledge and build on their existing skills.

Care assistants, even those with a great deal of practical experience, learn a great deal when gaining NVQ qualifications. This enables them to understand the problems older people face and equips them with the skills required to care for older people sensitively. This is good news for older people in homes, who benefit from higher quality care.

Many social services departments recognize the contribution that NVQ qualified staff make to the quality of care and are beginning to specify that a proportion of care assistants within each home should be either NVQ qualified or studying for NVQ qualifications. It is now government policy that 50% of all adults in practical occupations who do not have a recognized qualification should gain NVQ qualifications by the year 2000.

This book has been written specifically for the 100 000 care assistants working in nursing and residential homes who are studying for NVQ level 2 qualifications. It aims to supply care assistants and their managers with information and advice to help them meet the challenges of caring for older people in a rapidly changing environment. It provides:

- an understanding of how older people feel about homes
- an understanding of how age affects the body and mind
- information on how illness affects older people's abilities
- ways in which staff can work to help older people enjoy life
- basic knowledge on the legal rights of older people
- a guide to resources available to help carers to care for older people as individuals
- guidance on good practice within care homes.

Older people have the same feelings, fears and hopes as all adults. The aim of this book is to enable carers to communicate with older people to discover their needs and to work with individual older people to provide the best possible care.

Linda Nazarko

Acknowledgements

Producing this book would not have been possible without the co-operation and help of many people. I would like to thank my colleagues and the residents of Purley View who posed for the photographs in this book. My husband Ed who took most of the photographs. Grahame Jones who produced the illustrations.

   I would also like to thank the following companies who provided photographs and illustrations:

Simcare, The Coloplast Foundation, KCI Mediscus, Molnyke, Convatec, ArjoMechanaids, HNE Huntleigh, Parker Baths and Smith & Nephew.

Thanks to Lisa Field for believing in me: Sue Moore and Brenda Ross for their meticulous editing and helpful suggestions.

Thanks to Rumi Sethna – my long suffering employer.

And last, but not least, thanks to Rachael Nazarko, my daughter, and her friend Bubbles.

How to Use This Book

The National Vocational Qualifications are made up of elements or units. Reading this book as a whole will enable students to gain a greater understanding about the physical and psychological aspects of ageing. Each chapter relates to part of the NVQ level 2 course. Students studying for a particular unit will find most of the information on that subject in a particular chapter of the book.

A list of units/elements and the relevant chapters is given below.

Unit/element		Chapter
Z7c	Assist the client to prevent and minimize adverse effects of pressure	10
Z9	**Enable clients to maintain their personal hygiene and appearance**	**11**
Z9a	Enable clients to maintain personal cleanliness	11
Z9b	Support clients in personal grooming and dressing	11
Z10	**Enable clients to eat and drink**	**12**
Z10a	Enable clients to choose appropriate food and drink	12
Z10b	Enable clients to prepare for eating and drinking	12
Z10c	Assist clients with eating and drinking	12
Z11	**Enable clients to access and use toilet facilities**	**13**
Z11a	Enable clients to access toilet facilities	13
Z11b	Assist clients to use toilet facilities	13
Z11c	Collect and dispose of client's body waste	13

Z19   Enable clients to achieve physical comfort

Z19a   Assist in minimizing client discomfort and pain

Z19b   Assist in providing conditions to meet the client's need for rest

Dealt with throughout book. Chapters 3, 8, 9 and 10 particularly relevant

Chapter 1

Equality

Introduction

This chapter will examine and discuss:

- the role older people have in our society today
- the legal rights of the older person living in a home
- the rights to health care and services
- the right to be treated with dignity and respect; dignity and respect are so important that the whole book contains material on this issue
- confidentiality – discussed in greater detail in Chapter 7
- the rights of older people to make choices about how they choose to lead their lives; choice is one of the most important issues in caring for older people so this issue will recur throughout the book
- information to help the carer provide care appropriate to the older person's cultural background
- details of how carers can help people continue to attend church and practice their religion are given

Older people and society

In the past it was unusual for people to live as long as they do now. At the beginning of the century when old age pensions were introduced few older people lived long enough to collect their pensions. During this century improved living conditions and improved medical care have resulted in people living longer than before (Fig. 1.1).

As you can see in Fig. 1.1, the number of people over the age of 85 will have risen from 70 000 at the beginning of the century to 1.2 million by the end of the century. Most people living in homes are women. Statistics show that for every 77 women over the age of 85 years there are 23 men. Statistics also show that older men are less likely to be admitted to homes than women. When men are admitted to homes they require much greater levels of care than women. There are several reasons for this. Women in the past tended to marry men who were on average five years older.

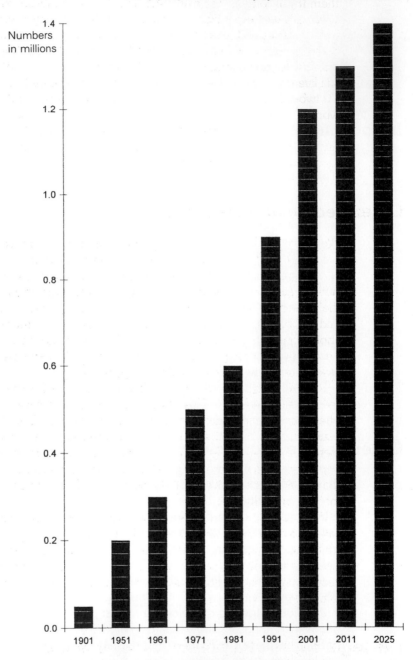

Fig. 1.1 Graph showing people aged 85 and over in the UK population from 1901 to 2025 (Source: Mortality Statistics Serial Tables 1841–1988. Office of Population Censuses and Surveys, London (1991)).

When these men become ill and require care, their wives care for them for as long as possible. Research shows that these younger wives are well organized and obtain help from family members, district nurses and social services so that the married older man is cared for at home for as long as possible. It is only when the older man's wife can no longer cope that he is admitted to care. Women still live on average five years longer than men and by the age of 70 two-thirds of all women are widowed or divorced. Half of the women over the age of 60 either had no children or have lived longer than their children. So women, because they live longer and married older men, are less likely to have anyone to care for them when they require help.

Older people and their families

We often hear people complaining that families no longer care for old people in the way that they did in the past. In fact few families cared for older people in the past because there were fewer older people. At the beginning of the century families often lived under the same roof. The family might consist of grandparents, parents and children. In many cases the family did not live together out of choice but because they could not afford separate homes. As people have become more prosperous it has become rare for several generations to live under the same roof.

Research, though, shows that families still care for the older members of the family. This research confirms what many people often forget – that older people have more experience and offer younger members of the family advice and support, while younger members of the family help with physical tasks which the older person may now find difficult. There are seven million carers in the UK. Many have given up their own well-paid jobs to care for a member of their family.

Research shows that families do provide practical help and support for older people. Carers can help families remain involved when the person is admitted to a home; further details are given in Chapter 4. Some older people do not have any family and because they may not have help and support they are more likely to be admitted to homes.

The legal rights of a person living in a home

A person living in a home has the same legal rights as any other citizen. In the USA there is a written constitution and every citizen is aware of their rights because these are written down. People being cared for in hospitals and homes have a series of basic rights which are legally binding. In the UK our legal system is older and has evolved over more than a thousand years. There is no legal declaration of each citizen's rights, but instead a series of Acts of Parliament and also common law which define a person's rights.

People living in homes have not given up any of their rights when they enter the home. If the person wishes to leave the home, staff cannot forcibly detain the person except in special circumstances. If the person is at serious risk of injuring themselves or others then a doctor, social worker or policeman can exercise special powers to detain the person for a limited period. If this is the case, the person will be transferred to hospital for care by nurses specializing in caring for people with mental health needs. Consent must be obtained before care is carried out or medication is given. Forcing a person to bath against her will or forcing a person to take medication or have treatment is an offence. Sensitive care will involve working with the older person to meet needs, not imposing a regime upon the individual.

Rights to health care and services

People living in homes have the same rights to health care as people living in their own homes. Older people have the same right to choose their own *general practitioner* (GP) as other adults. Most homes have a GP who visits the home on a regular basis and provides care for many of the older people living in the home. If the older person lives locally her GP can continue to visit and offer medical care. Unfortunately many older people admitted to homes are no longer in the area where the GP has agreed to provide care.

GPs may be unable to care for people who have moved out of the area in which they practice because of the difficulty in travelling some distance to visit the older person in the home. In most homes the older person moving out of the area to the home is asked if she wishes to receive medical care from the GP who visits the home. The person has the right to choose another GP in the local area if she wishes. In practice this can be difficult as some GPs are reluctant to offer care to individuals living in homes. Some GPs state that older people living in homes require more care than older people living in their own homes and prefer not to offer this service. If an older person does not wish to have care from the home's GP and a local GP cannot be found to offer care, then the older person, the family or the manager will have to contact the local Family Services Health Association (FSHA), who will find a GP in these circumstances. The number of the FSHA is in the telephone directory.

People living in homes have the same right to see *nurse specialists* as people living in their own homes. In some parts of the country people living in homes have received excellent specialist care from nurses specialising in areas such as diabetes, continence promotion, wound care and stoma care. In other parts of the country the creation of National Health Trusts has resulted in some older people finding it difficult to obtain these services. In some parts of the country trusts introduced charges for such care. If the older person or the home was unable or unwilling to pay those charges the person did not receive that care. Recently the government issued new guidance which stated clearly that such charges are illegal.

People living in homes are entitled to services such as *chiropody* and *physiotherapy*. Unfortunately although the number of people living in homes has increased tenfold since the mid-1980s the number of people employed to provide such service has not increased. In many areas staff working in homes find it difficult to obtain these services for patients. The local NHS trust has a responsibility to provide services for local people. If these services are not available your manager can inform the local *Community Health Council* (CHC) which monitors the performance of NHS trusts and can make senior members of the trust aware of the problems. The telephone number of the CHC will be in the local telephone book.

People suffering from incontinence who live in residential homes are normally supplied with *incontinence pads*. These pads are paid for by the local NHS trust. In most areas the district nurse visits and determines if pads are required. The nurse will then inform the NHS trusts and a certain number of pads are supplied for that person every month. If you work in a home run by social services the pads will usually be delivered to the home. If you work in a residential home run by either a charity or a private concern the pads will usually have to be collected. Pads are not supplied to people living in nursing homes. Here the pads must be purchased by the home and supplied to older people who require them.

Confidentiality

When an older person enters a home carers get to know the person's innermost secrets. The carer may, because of the nature of the caring relationship, know more about the person's thoughts and feelings than even the person's family. People who confide their secrets and share their feelings with carers do so because they trust carers completely and have confidence in the carer. The carer must guard those secrets well and maintain the person's trust.

In some homes, and also in hospital, sensitive information is bandied about. If a person suffers from diabetes this may be recorded on a label above the bed! In some homes charts giving details of the person's continence are displayed in corridors and lounge areas where other patients, relatives and even people delivering supplies can see them. If the older person suffers from haemorrhoids (piles) she could be deeply embarrassed if a carer mentioned this in front of another patient, even one who is sharing a room. Carers should be tactful and ensure that details of a personal nature are not discussed in front of others. This would not only be insensitive but also a breach of confidentiality. Confidentiality of information is dealt with in detail in Chapter 7.

Dignity and respect

All people have a right to be treated with dignity and respect. We all choose to work in a caring setting because we wish to care for people. Sometimes though something goes wrong and carers become insensitive to the person's need to be treated with dignity and respect. We have all heard of cases where people are placed on commodes in full view of others; of cases where people are not dressed properly and care is poor.

Sometimes carers ask: 'What is acceptable and what isn't? How do I know if the care I am giving is good enough?' The answer to this is simple. If the carer would be happy to be treated in such a way, if she would be happy for her own mother to be treated in this way, then the care is acceptable. If the carer would not be happy to be treated as her patients are treated then the care is unacceptable.

Choices

Older people living in homes have the same rights to make choices as people living within their own homes. Unfortunately it is much more difficult for people living within homes to exercise choice. People living in homes rely on staff to help them and many fear that if they complain they will be seen as 'trouble-makers' or 'moaners', and so many fit in and go along with the routine in the home. If older people do not make choices about how to lead their lives they can quickly lose all sense of control over their own lives. They become disinterested in their surroundings, and physical and mental health deteriorates.

Research shows that in homes where staff work hard to enable older people to remain involved in decisions about their day to day life, staff and patients are more fulfilled. Regular meetings between patients and staff help older people remain involved. In some homes patients have formed residents committees. These committees may plan recreational activities and in some homes they sit on panels to interview new members of staff.

Caring for older people from different cultural backgrounds

We live in a multicultural society, yet few people from ethnic minority groups live in homes. There are thought to be two reasons for this. First, many people who came to this country to work are only now reaching the age when they may require care in homes. Second, care within homes is geared to the native population. Older people entering homes feel vulnerable and anxious. People who have difficulty in speaking English and who have a different diet or religion may feel terrified by the thought of entering a home. In some areas homes have been set up specially to cater for people from certain religious or ethnic groups. Special homes have been set up to meet the needs of people from Poland, Italy, Germany and Hong Kong, and there is also a special home to care for Jewish people.

From time to time homes care for people from different cultures. If the person does not speak English, it can be difficult to communicate; further details on communication are given in Chapter 2. Care given should be appropriate to the person's needs. The person should, like all other patients, be treated in accordance with her culture and wishes. The diet should be appropriate to the person's culture; this is dealt with in detail in Chapter 12.

The person should be encouraged and helped to follow her chosen religion. People of different faiths celebrate special events. People of the Jewish faith celebrate the Passover. People of the Muslim faith celebrate Eid. People of the Hindu faith celebrate Diwali (the Hindu festival of light). People of different faiths should be encouraged to celebrate special festivals either with their family or with other patients in the home. With a little planning the home's calendar of celebrations can begin with New Year's Day and include St David's day, St Patrick's day, St George's day and all the other celebrations within a year.

Spiritual needs

People of all ages find that spirituality and religion play an important part in their lives. Many older people enjoy watching the Sunday service on television and appreciate the effort that staff have made to ensure that the minister visits. Many, though, would prefer, given a choice, to attend church. There is a great difference between listening to a service and taking part in one. Wherever possible the staff at the home should help older people who wish to attend church services to do so. The local ministers of religion can often put staff in touch with active church members who will escort the individual to church. Church members can befriend older people new to the area and help involve them in all types of church activities.

People who are not of the Christian faith also enjoy participating in religious services. Ministers and members of the Jewish, Muslim, Hindu and other faiths can help arrange transport so that, wherever possible the person can attend religious services.

Conclusion

Older people have the same rights as anyone else to be treated with dignity and respect and in a way which is appropriate to their cultural background. Ensuring that people are treated in this way at all times is vitally important. Many homes have policies which emphasize and reinforce the importance of this.

Portfolio preparation

- Some homes have defined their philosophy of care and this usually includes a statement about equality. Obtain a copy of this if your home has one.
- Some homes also have an operations policy. This normally gives details of how the home is to be run in order to fulfil its stated aim or philosophy. If your home has one include this in your portfolio.
- Check to see if your home has a policy on dignity and respect. Photocopy this and include it in your portfolio.
- If your home cares for people of different cultural backgrounds make notes on how their cultural and spiritual needs are met.

Further reading

Counsel & Care (1992) *Not Such Private Places*. Counsel & Care, London. This book examines issues relating to privacy and dignity in nursing and residential homes.

Chapter 2

Communicating

Introduction

> This chapter will:
>
> - explain the barriers to communication which are caused by physical disabilities
> - discuss the particular problems facing stroke patients
> - explain the types of communication problems stroke patients face
> - outline the problems people with Parkinson's disease face
> - discuss the different types of deafness
> - explain how to help older people use hearing aids
> - explain how confusion and dementia can cause communication problems
> - Give information and guidance to enable carers to communicate more effectively

Communicating with others

The ability to understand others and to make ourselves understood is a skill we often take for granted. In some circumstances, perhaps on holiday abroad, we have difficulty in communicating with others. Ending up with the wrong meal, being directed to the wrong place or being thought a little crazy by the locals is often part of the fun of being on holiday. Sometimes, though, having difficulty in communicating can be maddening.

Older people living in nursing and residential homes often have difficulty in understanding what carers are saying. If an older person does not understand what has been said then the reply can be inappropriate. The carer may think that the older person is confused. Some older people understand what the carer has said but have difficulty in making themselves understood.

Older people who have difficulty in understanding others or making themselves understood can react in different ways. Some can become frustrated, angry and aggressive, whilst others can become withdrawn and depressed. The ability to communicate is very important. Sometimes, because of illness, older people can have great difficulty in communicating their needs. Carers who are aware of the reasons why older people may have difficulty in communicating can use a range of skills to remove barriers which prevent communication.

Barriers to communicating with older people

Older people are admitted to nursing and residential homes because it is no longer possible to provide the care required at home. The majority of older people living in nursing and residential homes are in their eighties and nineties. Most older people, even of this age, continue to live at home. Those who enter nursing and residential homes do so because they are too infirm to continue living at home; some patients are physically frail but very alert, some are physically well but confused, while others are both physically and mentally frail. Most older people do not wish to leave their own homes and live in 'a home'. Older people admitted to homes often feel anxious and upset because of the move. They may become withdrawn and unwilling to communicate. Carers who take time getting to know the older person and encouraging the individual to express her feelings make an important contribution to her care.

How physical disabilities can affect the ability to communicate

Physical disabilities can affect the individual's ability to communicate in a number of ways. Strokes can affect the ability to understand speech and to speak. Parkinson's disease can cause individuals to have difficulty forming words and speech can sound slurred. People who are deaf may be unable to hear clearly, even when wearing a hearing aid. Hearing aids amplify all sound and background noise can make it difficult to hear clearly. Hearing aids can also make speech sound distorted, and so difficult to understand.

Communication and stroke patients

How strokes affect the ability to communicate

Strokes can cause communication problems if they affect the speech centre in the brain. In some cases older people do not understand what we are saying – it is as if we were speaking a foreign language. These people cannot receive and make sense of the messages we send them in our speech; this is known as *receptive dysphasia*.

There are degrees of dysphasia. People with *mild dysphasia* understand most of what is being said. Tiredness, background noise, people speaking too quickly or more than one person speaking at once affect their ability to understand. People with *moderate dysphasia* find it more difficult to follow conversations: long and complicated sentences are difficult to follow; some words are only partly understood. The individual may have difficulty concentrating and may be able to understand the start of a conversation but become confused if the conversation is too long. People with *severe dysphasia* may have difficulty in understanding even single words.

Many people who suffer from dysphasia after a stroke find that their condition gradually improves over weeks and months. People who are suffering from receptive dysphasia rely on tone of voice, movement and gestures to help fill in the words which they do not understand. Carers should ensure that older people who need glasses are wearing them, as this will help the dysphasic person to 'hear' and communicate.

Some individuals understand every word and gesture but cannot find the right words to communicate. They mix up words and may say 'yes' instead of 'no' or 'plate' instead of 'cup'. Some individuals have difficulty in finding the correct word and use a similar word instead. This difficulty in finding the correct word is known as *anomia* and is part of a general difficulty in expressing what they want to say. This is known as *expressive dysphasia*.

Strokes can affect the muscles of the throat, tongue, lips and face. Some older people have difficulty in swallowing after a stroke. Many older people wear dentures and these are kept in place partly by the muscles in the mouth. If these muscles are affected, dentures can slip around or be almost impossible to wear. Poor muscle control and difficulty with dentures can make it difficult for individuals to form words. This difficulty in articulating is known as *dysarthria*.

Some individuals lose the ability to speak. This is known as *aphasia*.

Reading and writing

Strokes can affect the vision; often individuals can only see out of half of each eye, which makes it difficult to read. This is known as *hemienopia*. It is important that older people who have worn glasses before a stroke continue to wear glasses following the stroke. Strokes can change the vision and an eye test can be arranged to see if new glasses are required. Sometimes words make no sense to an individual; this may improve in the weeks and months after a stroke.

Strokes can paralyse limbs and can cause individuals to lose the ability to write. Some older people can learn to write with a non-affected hand. Speech and language therapists can assess individuals with such problems and can help them to regain skills.

How carers can help

It is important to realise that many people can recover most if not all speech following a stroke. Recovery is dependent on the severity of the stroke, therapy from speech therapists, the individual's motivation and the help carers give. Carers can really make a difference and can help older people to recover or cope with communication problems after a stroke.

In many areas people who have suffered a stroke are invited to a 'stroke club'. These are normally held in local community health centres once or twice each week. The stroke club offers physiotherapy and exercise which help some stroke patients recover strength and movement to weakened or paralysed limbs. In other cases exercise helps prevent deformity which often develops if paralysed limbs are not moved and exercised. Speech therapy is also offered, normally consisting of individual and group speech therapy. Many people who suffer from strokes begin to recover speech but are conscious that their speech sounds slurred and strange at first. Speaking to others with similar problems at a stroke club helps individuals gain confidence. Carers are often asked to escort older people to stroke clubs, and some are asked to remain with the individual during the session.

Golden rules to help stroke patients communicate

- speak slowly
- use simple clear language
- use short sentences
- only ask one question at a time
- only give one piece of information at a time
- use gestures
- encourage the individual to use gestures
- encourage the individual to speak
- ensure that the individual who requires glasses is wearing them
- ensure that the individual who requires a hearing aid is wearing it.
- listen and be patient

Further information

Action for Dysphasic Adults
1 Royal Street
London SE1 7LL.
Telephone 0171 261 9572

This is a charity which provides information to dysphasic people, their carers and professionals. It produces a number of booklets which are supplied free to professionals, carers and dysphasic people. These include:

> *Lost for Words*, a general booklet about dysphasia
> *Stroke and Dysphasia*, a simple diagrammatic booklet
> *How to Help the Dysphasic Person*

>> (1)   In the early stages
>> (2)   With comprehension and speech
>> (3)   With reading and writing
>> (4)   With total communication
>> (5)   Complicating factors with dysphasia

Action for Dysphasic Adults also publish a number of books. *Living After a Stroke* by Diana Law is a personal account of a woman's struggle to overcome the effects of her stroke and may be of particular interest to carers. It may be available in your local or college library.

Parkinson's disease

Parkinson's disease is a disorder of the brain. Disorders affecting the brain are referred to as neurological diseases or disorders. Parkinson's disease is a progressive neurological disease. It is caused by a reduction in *dopamine*. Dopamine enables nerve cells to transmit messages to each other. An individual suffering from Parkinson's disease has difficulty in moving because of the disease. The disease also affects the ability to move the muscles in the mouth and tongue which are used to form words. Individuals suffering from Parkinson's disease often have difficulty in speaking clearly and their words can become slurred.

The disease is now treated with a number of drugs which help replace the dopamine shortage which causes the disease. At first the individual with Parkinson's disease appears to have fully recovered because of the medication. As the disease progresses greater amounts of medication are required. Individuals in the early stages of Parkinson's disease are normally able to live at home. It is only in the later stages of the disease that they are admitted to nursing and residential homes.

At this stage many older people suffering from Parkinson's disease are taking large amounts of two or more drugs to control the disease. These drugs work for shorter and shorter periods and in the final stages of the disease one of these drugs may be given as often as every three hours while the individual is awake.

Individuals who have Parkinson's disease may be able to speak clearly if they have recently had some medication but as the medication begins to wear off they may have great difficulty in forming words. Sometimes the drugs given to control Parkinson's disease can cause the individual to hallucinate or become confused.

Golden rules to help patients with Parkinson's disease communicate

- Speak slowly and clearly
- Give the individual time to speak
- Be aware that ability to speak will vary
- Be patient
- Check that you have understood what has been said
- Encourage the individual to speak

How deafness affects the individual's ability to communicate

Hearing loss is often referred to as the 'hidden handicap'. It is very common; an estimated 7.5 million people in the UK have some degree of hearing loss. It is estimated that 4 million of these would benefit from hearing aids but only 2.5 million actually have one. Hearing deteriorates as people age and by the age of 70, approximately 60% of people have hearing loss. This figure rises to 90% by the age of 90 years.

As the majority of people living in nursing and residential homes are in their 80s and 90s, most of them will suffer from hearing loss. This affects their ability to understand and respond to carers and to others living in the home. Unfortunately many people who come in contact with deaf people automatically dismiss them as stupid. Older people with hearing loss state that others are inclined to 'talk over them' and that people who are deaf 'tend to get left out of conversations'. Other people are 'inclined to think that deaf people are not with it'.

Many older people with hearing loss find communicating with others extremely frustrating and if they feel that people are ignoring them, talking over them or treating them as though they were senile, they may simply give up trying to communicate. As one lady with hearing loss stated: 'If they make no effort why should I bother?' Carers who understand the causes and effects of deafness will be able to communicate more effectively with older people with hearing loss, and can encourage them to communicate and take part in the daily life of the home.

Causes of hearing loss

Wax

The commonest cause of hearing loss is wax in the ears. Even older people who suffer from deafness find that their hearing is improved if a build-up of wax in the ear is removed. Older people who appear to be deaf should have their ears checked by a doctor who will use an instrument known as an *auroscope* to check for the presence of wax in the ear. Normally any wax in the ear is softened by putting drops in one or both ears three times daily for up to five days Carers in residential home may be asked to put these drops in an older person's ears. The ears are then normally syringed by a qualified nurse in nursing homes. In residential homes the district nurse may visit to syringe the ears.

The qualified nurse will often ask the carer to help with this procedure. The older person is seated in a chair and the procedure explained. Normally tap water is heated to body temperature (37°C) and drawn up in a metal syringe designed specially for syringing ears. The assistant places a plastic sheet and then a towel around the older person's shoulders and neck. The nurse squirts water from the syringe into the ear at an angle; the water trickles out of the ear and is caught in a kidney shaped dish by the assistant. The syringing washes the softened wax out of the ear and it is collected with the water in the dish. This can be repeated if the nurse finds that not all the wax has been removed.

The doctor normally checks that the ears are clear of wax on the next visit to the home. If hearing is still not normal then the doctor will consider that the individual is suffering from hearing loss and will arrange a hearing test at the local hospital. Hearing tests are known as *audiograms* and cannot be carried out if ears are full of wax.

Conductive deafness

Conductive deafness is caused by damage or obstruction to the structure of the ear. Wax in the ear, by blocking the ear, can cause conductive deafness, and hearing is restored when the wax is removed. A heavy cold can cause the ears to become blocked and can cause temporary conductive deafness. An ear infection, which if untreated can persist for months or years, can cause conductive deafness. A perforated ear drum can cause deafness; a repair of the perforation can restore hearing.

Sensory neural deafness

Although sensory neural deafness is the most common in older people, there is no treatment available. As adults age the nerve which connects the ear to the brain, the auditory nerve, becomes less sensitive to noise, and the ability to hear is reduced. Hearing is lost first at higher frequencies. This means that older people with hearing difficulties can hear low pitched noise quite well but have difficulty with higher pitched sounds. Women tend to speak at a higher pitch than men and many older people find it more difficult to follow a woman's speech than that of a man. The only available treatment for sensory neural deafness is to make sounds louder so that the individual can hear. Hearing aids are used to amplify sounds so that people with sensory neural deafness can hear.

Hearing aids

If an older person has difficulty hearing, their GP writes a letter to the ear, nose and throat specialist at the local hospital. The older person visits the hospital as an outpatient and hearing is tested. The type of deafness and causes are identified. If the individual is suffering from sensory neural deafness arrangements are normally made for a hearing aid to be supplied.

Hearing aids consist of two main parts. The ear piece, which is made of clear plastic, fits into the ear. Each ear piece is made specially for the individual. A mould of the ear is taken and the ear piece is made to fit snugly into the ear. A tube connects the ear piece to the amplifier section of the aid. The amplifier section is normally known as 'the body' of the aid. The body is mass pro-duced. Most older people who are supplied with NHS hearing aids are supplied with an aid which fits behind the ear. People who are extremely deaf may be supplied with a different type of aid which has an earpiece attached to a long cord. The body of the aid is the size of a pocket calculator and is clipped onto the chest over clothing.

Encouraging and helping older people to use their hearing aids

Many older people who have been supplied with hearing aids no longer use them. This is known as 'fruit bowl syndrome' because older people often leave their unused hearing aids in fruit bowls. In one survey of nursing and residential homes, half of the older people who had hearing aids did not wear them. The reasons given were that they found them difficult to put in and adjust or that the aids no longer worked.

Older people living in homes often find it difficult to perform tasks which require fine muscle control. They find it difficult to do up small buttons, and similar tasks. This may be because of illness. Arthritis can leave fingers stiff, Parkinson's disease can cause a tremor. In most cases older people do not ask carers for help: 'they have enough to do'. Ear pieces must be fitted firmly into the ear if the aid is to work. Aids must be turned on and turned on the correct setting. The setting varies from individual to individual and environment to environment but is set at the level which enables the older person to hear easily. Batteries must be changed regularly. These simple tasks take only a few minutes but enable older people to communicate with carers and others. This saves time and reduces frustration throughout the day.

Helping people with hearing aids to hear

Many people, including some qualified staff, think that if an older person has a hearing aid they can hear normally. Unfortunately this is not the case. A hearing aid works by amplifying all sound and aids can easily distort hearing. Carers communicating with older people who have hearing loss, including those who wear hearing aids, should use special techniques to make it easier for individuals to understand them. These include:

- Cut down on background noise. Close the door if it is noisy outside. Close the window to reduce the roar of traffic.
- Move near to the person.
- Speak a little more loudly than usual – but don't shout. Shouting can appear threatening. It also distorts the voice, raising the pitch and making it more difficult for the person to hear.
- Always face the person.
- Speak directly to the person. Do not attempt to have conversations with more than one person at the same time. The deaf person will have difficulty following this.
- Do not cover your mouth whilst speaking.
- Speak slowly and clearly.
- If you have not been understood, rephrase the sentence using different words with similar meanings.
- Check that the individual has understood.
- Use gestures.
- Offer to write things down.

Communicating with deaf people who do not have hearing aids

Hearing aids can only help people who have some hearing. Some deaf people are totally deaf and are not helped by hearing aids. In this situation carers must find other ways to communicate. Many profoundly deaf older people have learnt to lip read. If this is the case the carer should use the techniques mentioned above.

Some older people do not have hearing aids because they are waiting for an appointment for one to be fitted. It can take six months to obtain an appointment to see the ear, nose and throat specialists at many hospitals. It can take a further three months to obtain a hearing aid. In these circumstances the carer can write things down for the older person. It can be helpful to supply a notebook and pen which the older person carries. Carers can then write down messages and the older person can reply. Remember to write clearly. If the older person's eyesight is poor, writing in large letters can help.

Further information

The British Association of the Hard of Hearing (Hearing Concern)
7–11 Armstrong Road
London W3 7JL.
Telephone 0181 743 1110

This organisation operates a scheme known as the sympathetic hearing scheme. This aims to make people more aware of hearing difficulties. It produces leaflets, and a video that can be hired, which allows carers to understand what speech sounds like to hearing aid wearers. The association is run by people who are hard of hearing. It has a network of volunteers and may be able to provide a volunteer speaker to visit the nursing or residential home where you work, or your college, to speak to a group of carers. The association also produces a magazine four times a year.

The British Deaf Association (BDA)
38 Victoria Place
Carlisle
Cumbria CA1 1HU.
Telephone 01228 48844

This is an organization for deaf people. It produces a monthly newsletter as well as information sheets and leaflets.

The Royal National Institute for Deaf People (RNID)
105 Gower Street
London WC1E 6AH.
Telephone 0171 387 8033

The RNID produces a guide to local and national services for deaf people, plus a range of useful leaflets including: *The Ear and How It Works*; and *Understanding Hearing Aids*.

Further Reading

Sound Barriers – A study of the needs of older people with hearing loss living in residential care and nursing homes. Available from the charity Council and Care, Twyman House, 16 Bonny Street, London NW1 9PG. Telephone 0171 485 1550.

Communicating with older people suffering from confusion

Communicating with older people who suffer from confusion is perhaps one of the greatest challenges that carers face. It is difficult and some carers feel that it is not worth trying because they will be unable to 'get through' to the individual. In many cases a little time and patience will pay dividends and carers will be able to communicate with the confused older person. The ability to do so enables the carer to meet the person's needs. People who have their needs met are more likely to be relaxed, settled and happy within the home. It is important that carers are aware of the causes of confusion as this will affect their approach to the individual.

Causes of confusion

There is always a reason for confusion. Often staff in homes assume that if someone becomes confused, 'It's just her age ... what do you expect at 92.' There are two major causes of confusion. The first is an acute illness. The second is that the individual is suffering from a neurological disease such as senile dementia.

Older people who have suddenly become confused are usually ill. People who have a chest infection or a urine infection often become confused. Carers often know patients better than trained staff because they spend more time with them. They can often observe a cough or notice that an older person's urine smells. They should inform nursing staff, and nursing and medical staff should investigate and treat.

Medication can cause confusion. Carers, because they spend a great deal of time with patients, are often the first to notice any side effects caused by medication. In residential homes care staff will be aware of any changes of medication because they are usually responsible for giving out medication. In nursing homes medication is given out by trained staff. Carers, though, are often aware that medication has been changed. Carers who notice that an individual has become confused should inform a qualified nurse in the nursing home and your manager or a senior member of staff in a residential home.

Sometimes confusion creeps up slowly but staff should always check that there is no treatable physical cause before accepting confusion. Certain diseases such as diabetes, Parkinson's disease, thyroid disease and kidney disease can cause confusion. The qualified nurse or doctor should be informed if an older person is becoming confused.

Mental illness and confusion

Many older people suffer from senile dementia. It is estimated that 25% of people over the age of 85 suffer from this mental illness. The commonest cause of dementia is *Alzheimer's disease*. This is a progressive mental illness. At first individuals become forgetful and muddled but eventually they become completely disorientated and unable to care for themselves. Individuals suffering from dementia are normally able to carry on living at home in the early stages of the disease. When the disease becomes more advanced they are admitted to residential and nursing homes. Normally individuals admitted to nursing homes are suffering from a more advanced stage of dementia than those in residential homes. Dementia is a progressive neurological disease which eventually leads to death.

Memory loss
Memory is lost in dementia. Short-term memory is most affected. The individual suffering from dementia may not be able to remember what he or she ate at lunchtime but can remember the events of long ago very clearly. It is important that the carer bears this in mind. An older person with Alzheimer's disease can often remember the names of close friends and family but forgets the carers' names. He or she may have to be shown the way back to the bedroom each time because short-term memory is so poor. People suffering from Alzheimer's disease can become very bewildered because they cannot remember where they are. The carer has an important role to play in gently reminding the older person of his or her whereabouts.

Wandering, shouting and screaming

Many older people with Alzheimer's disease wander around without a purpose. They may shout out and scream. This is very distressing for carers and other patients. It is important to find out if there are reasons for the older person's behaviour:

- Is the patient in pain? If so pain killers may help.
- Is the patient constipated? Treatment will help.
- Is the patient hungry? Perhaps that walk to the kitchen is to get a snack.
- Is the patient bored? Spending time doing something with the patient will help.
- Does the patient want to go for a walk? Imagine how you would feel after a few weeks in the nursing home.

Making sense of an individual's behaviour

Often confused patients will do things which upset other patients, but if we take time to find out the reasons for the behaviour we can improve the situation. An elderly confused lady was upsetting all the other patients because she was constantly taking their hand-bags and hiding them in her locker. She had no family or visitors. The care assistant looking after her brought in a handbag from home, put a comb, some lipstick, tissues and a few biscuits in the bag. The lady stopped taking other people's bags because she had one of her own.

Carers can, by taking time to talk to and listen to the older person, help them enjoy a good quality of life within the home. Carers should communicate their findings to more senior staff within homes so that they can be recorded and all staff are aware of information which improves care.

Golden rules for communicating with confused people

- Eliminate any distractions. Find a quiet place to speak to the confused person
- Take time to communicate. Sit down and relax. If you appear hurried or harassed the individual may become tense.
- Speak slowly and clearly.
- Use plain language.
- Use short sentences.
- Only use one idea in each sentence.
- Do not give too many choices in one sentence. For example ask, 'Would you like a bath?' Not 'Would you like a bath or would you prefer to wash?'

- Ask the patient's family what methods of communication they found most effective.
- Spend time with the patient.
- If you suspect there are other barriers to communication, such as deafness or poor eyesight, inform a trained nurse within the nursing home or your manager or a senior member of staff in the residential home, so that the individual can be helped, perhaps by having a hearing aid or new glasses.

Communicating with people who do not speak English

Some older people have come to the UK from abroad and have never learnt to speak English. Many other older people have learnt to speak English but because of a neurological condition such as a stroke or dementia have lost the ability to communicate in English. Many people understand more of a language than they can speak. The older person's family can help you to discover how much the person understands. Carers can rule a piece of paper into two columns and write words in English on one side; the older person's family and friends can write these words in the person's own language in the other column and this can be used to help communicate. A scrapbook full of pictures with the words written in English and the person's own language can help. Using a picture board, such as those used by stroke patients, can also help with communication.

Beware of using gestures. Before you use gestures check with the person's family that the gestures you use have the same meaning in that person's culture. If gestures are the same then use them. If gestures differ slightly, make a note of this. When it is important that staff and patient communicate accurately, perhaps when the person is feeling unwell or is attending an outpatient's appointment, ask if a member of the family can act as an interpreter. Finally don't forget that facial expressions and touch are very important aids to understanding. Face the person so that you can be seen clearly and use touch to reinforce your words. It is important to sit down if the individual is seated. Getting down to the same level makes communication friendlier, less threatening and easier.

Portfolio preparation

- Gather information from the sources mentioned in this chapter. This information can be used as part of your portfolio preparation

■ Collect information on an older person whom you care for who has difficulty in communicating. Outline the reasons for this difficulty and give details of ways in which the person is helped to communicate.

Chapter 3

Abuse

Introduction

Abuse of older people was first recognized 25 years ago but even today few homes have specific policies that prevent abuse from occurring and outline action to be taken in the event of abuse. This chapter gives information on:

- the different types of abuse including:
  - physical abuse
  - passive abuse
  - abuse of medications
  - psychological abuse
  - financial abuse
- the factors which increase the likelihood of abuse
- how to identify the patients most at risk of abuse
- warning signs of abuse
- action to take if abuse is occurring in your home
- the legal rights of older people living in homes
- caring for confused patients
- caring for patients who wander
- coping with older people who shout and scream
- caring for people who are aggressive

What is abuse?

There are many definitions of abuse:

'A single or repeated act occurring within a relationship where there is an expectation of trust, which causes harm to an individual over the age of 65.'

'Abuse may range from a spontaneous act of frustration to the systematic terrorising of an older person.'

Elder abuse is mistreatment of an older person. It can, as the definitions show, be a single act or a long-term pattern of abuse. Abuse can have a long-term effect on the older person's physical and mental health. Many people when they hear the term abuse immediately think of physical abuse. There are a number of other types of abuse as well.

Physical abuse

Physical abuse ranges from deliberately hitting and hurting the older person through to neglect. The person abused may be hit or slapped. She may be handled roughly and may develop bruises on forearms and shins as a result. She may be pulled or pushed.

Passive abuse

Passive abuse is the term used when the older person's needs are neglected. Their needs may be unmet: the call bell may be 'dropped' on the floor out of the person's reach; the walking frame may be too far away for the person to reach it. These acts effectively cut the person off and prevent her from moving around or calling for help.

Aids which the older person depends on may be 'lost' or the person may not be able to reach them without help: without a hearing aid the person cannot hear; without glasses she may be unable to see, and without teeth she will have great difficulty eating. The individual may not be helped to wash or bathe. In some cases people are left in nightclothes during the day or dressed in shabby soiled clothing. The person who requires help to eat or drink may not receive it and may become dehydrated and ill as a result.

In many cases passive abuse occurs because carers have not received training and have not developed the skills required to help care for the older person.

Abuse of medications

Abuse of medications may occur where staff are unable to meet the person's needs and ask medical staff to prescribe sedatives. The older person who is wandering around the home upsetting other patients has a reason for wandering. Educated staff who are aware of this will try to find out the reason. The older person may be hungry, cold, searching for a book or a handbag, or may simply be bored. Giving them a sedative solves nothing. The person will continue to walk around because his needs remain unmet. Now, however, because he has been sedated he is at greater risk of falling and injuring himself. In many homes older people are given sleeping tablets each night. Is this for the benefit of the patients or the staff?

Psychological abuse

Psychological abuse is shouting, swearing, laughing at, humiliating, ignoring or frightening an older person. Psychological abuse can affect the older person to just as great an extent as physical abuse. Carers should be sensitive to the older person's feelings, as a thoughtless comment can cause great offence to an older person living in the home.

Financial abuse

Financial abuse is stealing an older person's money or belongings. The abuse may be carried out by a member of staff, a member of the family or a 'friend'. The older person may be duped into signing papers giving access to savings or property. She may be asked to give valuable jewellery to a carer, relative or 'friend' for safekeeping.

Older people who have their nursing home fees met by either the Department of Social Security (DSS) or the local council receive a 'personal allowance'. Prior to the introduction of the Community Care Act some patients agreed to spend part of this allowance on paying the home's fees if they were above DSS levels. When the Community Care Act was introduced in April 1993 Social Services Departments (SSDs) became responsible for paying for the care of people who had less than £8000 in savings. In most parts of the country SSDs made it clear, when entering into contracts with homes, that they would meet the home's fees and that the individual was to have their personal allowance to spend as he or she wished.

Under both DSS and SSD payment systems, the personal allowance is paid on a pension book. Many older people are unable to cash this personally at the local post office and rely on a relative to do this, or in some circumstances a senior member of staff at the home may do it. In some circumstances either relatives or staff members may defraud the older person of this money.

Sexual abuse

Sexual abuse is forcing an older person to take part in any sexual activity without consent.

Which patients are most at risk of abuse?

Abuse in caring situations has been recognized for some time. Abuse is rare in settings where people are alert. It occurs more frequently when staff are caring for people who are unable to protect themselves or to protest. Victims of abuse are often:

- Over 75 years old
- Female
- Physically dependent on staff

- Requiring high levels of care
- May have communication problems
- May be confused

Not all older people who are abused fit into the categories given above. Any older person is at risk of abuse. Research has shown that older people living in homes who require high levels of care are particularly at risk. Older people who are 'difficult' and whom staff find it a strain to care for are at risk. People who have communication problems are at greater risk of abuse than those who are able to complain.

Who abuses older people?

The person who abuses the older person is usually someone the older person knows well – a person who in normal circumstances, the older person could trust. Relatives may abuse the person during visits. This abuse can be physical or psychological. In some cases relatives can bring medication from home and give this to the older person. Sometimes relatives can persuade or intimidate the older person into signing over property or valuables or into giving away jewellery. 'Friends' may abuse the older person. A member of staff may abuse the older person, and could be anyone who comes into contact with them: a domestic, a carer or a registered nurse.

Possible signs that abuse is occurring

Recently the United Kingdom Central Council (UKCC), the body which regulates the professional conduct of registered nurses, issued a special report on the professional conduct of nurses working in nursing homes. The report expressed concern at the rapid increase in cases of abuse and neglect of older people living in these homes. In many cases the matron of the home stated that she was unaware that abuse was taking place until it was reported. Often if an individual is being abused there are warning signs. These include:

- a history of falls
- unexplained injuries or injuries where the description of the 'accident' and the injuries do not correspond
- the person is quiet and withdrawn
- the person is nervous and eager to please
- bruising, particularly to shins and forearms
- cuts and tears to skin

- poor hygiene –the person may be dirty and smelly
- poor diet – the person may be very undernourished and thin
- insufficient fluids – the person may be very dehydrated
- isolation – the person may be left in her room and may be unable to move out of it without help
- the person is unable to call for help as she has no access to a call bell
- aids are 'forgotten' or lost

Why abuse can occur in homes

Abuse within homes is completely unacceptable. It is more likely to occur in poorly managed homes; in homes where there are insufficient staff to meet older people's needs staff are under greater pressure. In some homes staff are expected to give care they have not been trained to give, and may find themselves 'out of their depth'. In other homes staff may feel that they cannot turn to registered nurses or their manager for help and advice. In some homes carers do not receive sufficient supervision.

Older people now living in nursing and residential homes are more acutely ill than before and require greater amounts of care. In some homes training and education programmes (such as NVQ courses) have been introduced. Abuse is more likely to occur in homes where staff feel overworked, unsupported, unable to cope and receive little training and education.

What to do if abuse occurs

In some situations the inexperienced carer may be unsure if an older person is being abused. The carer may witness a colleague appearing to argue with an older person but it may be that the colleague and the older person are teasing each other. In another situation the carer may feel that a colleague is refusing to help an older person, for example:

'Mary get a wheelchair and wheel me downstairs please . . .'
'Why don't you get your walking stick and I'll walk down with you Mr Blackburn . . .'

In this case the carer may be encouraging Mr Blackburn to maintain his independence and to continue walking. If you feel unsure in such situations you could ask the person who is with you. Many inexperienced carers who are new to the home do not wish to risk upsetting staff. Find someone in the home you can trust, perhaps the matron or manager and ask, 'Does Mr Blackburn

normally walk to the lounge?' You may discover that Mr Blackburn has come to the home for a period of convalescence, has lost
confidence in his ability to walk and needs support and encouragement.

In other cases, sadly the carer can be in no doubt that a colleague's behaviour is unacceptable and the older person is being
abused. You may be on a placement or may be a new member of
staff. You may fear that you will be seen as a trouble maker and
that you will suffer as a result of reporting the abuse. You cannot
ignore it – you **must** tell someone. The older person may be
unable to tell staff what is happening; they may be too frightened
to speak out. If you turn a blind eye the abuse will continue and
may get worse.

If you feel able to, ask to speak to the matron or manager and
discuss the situation. Action can then be taken. If you do not feel
able to approach the manager perhaps you could send a letter or
leave a note giving information about the situation. Even if you are
not able to sign the note at least you will have informed the
manager. If no action is taken or if you do not feel able to
approach the manager, you can contact the registration and
inspection unit for the home.

Nursing homes are inspected by the local health authority. If you
ring the local hospital they will give you the number of the registration unit. Residential homes are inspected by the registration and
inspection unit run by social services. If you ring the local town hall
they will give you the number of the unit. You can inform the
registration unit of your concerns; your call will be in complete
confidence and the inspection unit will take action. Even if you do
not wish to leave your name the call will still be treated seriously.

You can, if you prefer, inform the person's care manager of the
situation. Details of who the older person's care manager is should
be recorded in the person's records. You may wish to call a help-
line for advice and support. Details of these are given at the end of
the chapter.

Abuse – the legal position

It is unlawful to abuse a person. Criminal charges can be brought
against the abuser under the Offences Against the Person Act
1861. There are plans to update this law and the Law Commission recently issued a report recommending changes. If a registered nurse is accused of abuse the governing body for nursing
staff, the UKCC, conducts an investigation. When registered
nurses have been found guilty of abuse they are normally 'struck
off' the register and can no longer practice.

Preventing abuse

The way a home is managed can make abuse more or less likely to occur. In homes where older people are respected and treated with dignity and respect the possibility of abuse is reduced. In this atmosphere older people and their families will have developed a good relationship with the manager and staff and will be able to raise concerns. Listening to and communicating with older people individually and at regular patient meetings will help prevent abuse or detect it quickly.

A home where staff are supported and supervised will prevent staff from feeling 'useless', 'out of their depth' and reaching the end of their tether because they are unable to cope with certain situations. A programme of staff education and training helps all staff to develop a greater understanding of the needs of older people. An educational programme helps staff to feel valued, and increased knowledge leads to improved care. In many homes where older people have been neglected the main problem has been that the staff did not know how to meet the needs of older people. In homes where abuse has occurred staff morale is poor, many staff have had no training for many years and management has been ineffective.

The home should have a series of procedures in place which help to detect signs of abuse quickly. Each home is required to keep details of accidents – further details are given in Chapter 6. Every accident which occurs should be written in the accident book. If the home has a policy of reviewing accidents and investigating the reasons for them any abuse can be quickly detected, investigated and action taken. A record of any pressure sores which occur will quickly detect cases of poor care and neglect. A record of complaints and suggestions will help detect problems in the early stages.

Financial abuse

Financial abuse can occur. In many homes the older person keeps a small amount of money with them and money is held by the home for safekeeping. Staff can use this money to buy items such as toiletries or snacks for the patients. It is essential, if the home holds money for the individual's use, that complete records are kept of this. The record should give details of money received and spent. This record protects staff against allegations of financial abuse.

Occasionally relatives who collect the personal allowance for the older person fail to pass this money on to the individual and fail to supply items which the person requires, despite requests from staff. In the past, when fees were met from DSS funds, there was little that could be done in this situation as the DSS did not wish to be involved. Since the introduction of the Community Care Act the situation has changed. If staff at the home ask the relative either to purchase items or leave money for these and the relative refuses, social services will take action. If the staff suspect that the relative or 'friend' is stealing the personal allowance, this can be discussed with the manager of the home. The manager will discuss the situation with social services, and social services will investigate and take action to ensure that the older person receives a personal allowance.

Caring for older people who are confused

It is easy to label older people as confused. A few years ago a nurse who was studying for an elderly care qualification conducted a survey on how older people are treated. She went shopping and got on buses. When she lost her way and asked for help people were helpful. When she misheard people repeated what they had said. Then, wearing make-up and a wig so that she looked old, she did exactly the same things. People were less helpful and treated her as a confused old lady, not because of her behaviour but because of her age. As adults we are allowed to mishear or misunderstand or be absent minded, but older people who behave in the same way can quickly be labelled as confused.

People who have difficulty in communicating can easily be wrongly labelled as confused. The deaf person who understands only part of the conversation may be thought confused. The person who has suffered a stroke and who uses the wrong word may be thought of as confused. It is important that carers listen to the older person and make sure that the person is not having difficulty in communicating, before deciding that they are confused.

Causes of confusion

Confusion is not a disease, it is a symptom. The first sign of illness in many older people is that they become confused. If this happens the carer should ask that a professional nurse or doctor sees the patient to find out the cause of the confusion. It can be caused by either physical or mental illness. Many people who become confused will recover if the cause of the confusion is treated, but there is no treatment for dementia at present. Causes of confusion include:

■ chest infection
■ urine infection

- wound infection
- diabetes
- anaemia
- an imbalance of chemicals in the blood (electrolyte imbalance)
- medication
- head injury
- thyroid disease – a thyroid gland which is underactive produces less of the hormone thyroxine; a deficiency of this
  hormone slows the person down physically and mentally
- Parkinson's disease
- depression
- dementia
- dehydration

Treatment of physical causes of confusion

Infection can cause confusion. If the infection is caused by a virus (such as the 'flu virus), antibiotics will not help. Antibiotics are only effective in treating bacteria. There are two main types of bacteria, known as gram negative and gram positive because of their appearance under the microscope. Certain antibiotics are only effective in treating gram negative or gram positive bacteria. Other antibiotics are effective in treating diseases caused by both gram negative and gram positive bacteria; these are known as broad spectrum antibiotics.

In recent years more of the bacteria which cause infections in older people living in homes have become resistant to the more commonly used antibiotics. If the bacteria are resistant to the antibiotic, the antibiotic will not cure the infection. Many homes now have policies to prevent the spread of infection. These often include sending specimens to ensure that the correct antibiotic is used. The person with a suspected urine infection would have a specimen of urine sent to the microbiology laboratory, where the staff would check for the presence of infection and advise the doctor on the most effective antibiotic to use.

If diabetes is suspected, investigations will be carried out and treatment given. This may include either insulin injections or tablets or, if the diabetes is mild, a diabetic diet.

If thyroid disease is present a blood sample will be sent to check the level of thyroid hormone, and tablets containing the hormone thyroxine will be given if required.

If the person is thought to be suffering from Parkinson's disease the doctor will examine them and prescribe medication to treat the disease. This is usually very effective in the early stages of the disease.

If anaemia has caused confusion this will be investigated. Any disease which has caused the anaemia will be treated, iron tablets will normally be prescribed and the older person will be encouraged to eat a diet rich in iron.

An imbalance in the chemicals in the blood (known as electrolytes) can cause confusion. This imbalance may be caused by medication such as diuretic tablets, diarrhoea, over-use of laxatives or prolonged vomiting. Any imbalance will be treated.

If medication has caused the confusion the person's doctor will alter the medication. If head injury has caused confusion urgent hospital treatment will be required. If depression has caused the person to become confused the doctor may prescribe anti-depressant tablets.

Dementia may cause confusion. There is no cure for dementia at present.

Dementia

Dementia is the name used for a group of diseases affecting brain function. There are two main types: multi-infarct dementia and Alzheimer's disease.

Multi-infarct dementia

Multi-infarct dementia is thought to be responsible for 20% of all cases of dementia. A small clot interrupts the blood supply to an area of the brain, and this leads to the death of an area of brain tissue and is known as an infarction. Many of these small infarctions cause brain tissue to die and the person loses the ability to remember and reason.

Multi-infarct dementia is:

- More common in men, because it is a disease of the arteries supplying the brain. Men are more at risk of arterial disease than women, who are protected from the effects of arterial disease by female hormones which are produced until menopause. Women of the older generation are less likely to have smoked than men and smoking increases the risk of arterial disease.
- Often present in people who suffer from high blood pressure (hypertension).
- Often present in people who have other signs of arterial disease such as angina.
- Sufferers can deteriorate suddenly and then stay at that level until another brain infarction occurs.

Medical treatment aims to prevent or reduce the number of infarcts which will cause brain damage. If the person's blood pressure is high, this will be treated. If the person is overweight he should be encouraged to lose weight. If he smokes he should be encouraged to give up. If the person has arterial disease this will be treated by the doctor. Many people who suffer from multi-infarct dementia are prescribed a junior aspirin each day. Research has shown that this small dose of aspirin helps prevent blood clots forming and greatly reduces the risk of further brain infarction.

Alzheimer's disease

Alzheimer's disease is named after a German neurologist who first described the disease at the beginning of the century. The cause of Alzheimer's disease is not known. There have been many theories over the years but none have been proved. It is known that the number of people suffering from Alzheimer's disease increases with age. Research has shown that 25% of all people over the age of 85 suffer from dementia, and that 80% of those people suffer from Alzheimer's disease. Alzheimer's disease is:

- a gradual slow deterioration of mental function
- memory loss is the first sign
- the person has difficulty in learning new things
- old memories are retained – the person remembers family but may forget about the new grandchild who was born recently
- old skills and habits are retained
- the person can easily become lost in new places.

Caring for people suffering from dementia

Dementia is a progressive disease. People who suffer from it have a vast range of abilities. In the early stages of dementia the individual may be forgetful, have difficulty handling money or remembering what is for lunch. In the advanced stages, the individual may be unable to recognize her daughter or her own face in the mirror. She may be unable to wash, dress, use the toilet, feed herself or walk without a great deal of help from staff. Obviously the type of care required is very different, but the aims of care remain the same.

Some people who suffer from dementia cope well because they have a routine. This gives the day structure and they depend on this routine to help them cope. It is important, if a routine is established, that each carer maintains it. If the person normally has breakfast and then bathes, dresses and has coffee in her room, a change in the routine by the carer can cause the person to become confused and disorientated.

The older person should be treated with dignity and respect. Their preferred title should be used. A retired doctor may wish to be referred to as Dr Lawson and a retired headmistress may wish to be known as Miss Anderson. Carers who use first names to people who have been referred to all their lives by their titles, deprive the older person of dignity and respect and may increase confusion. The individual may forget to close the bathroom or toilet door. Carers should ensure that they remind the person and help maintain the person's dignity.

It is easy for staff to see all confused older people as lacking in personality and to treat all people with dementia in the same way. Staff should aim to care for the individual. If the person is unable to express preferences, relatives and friends can often tell staff about the person's preferences. The woman who liked to have her hair permed and set should be encouraged and helped to maintain her usual hairstyle. The woman who preferred to wear trousers and blouses should not be discouraged from wearing these clothes because dresses are 'easier'. The person who detests fish and who is unable to request an alternative should have this noted so that she does not refuse lunch and go hungry or spend the afternoon trying to get into the kitchen to find some food. People suffering from dementia are often able to continue to perform activities which they have been doing for decades, such as washing or dressing, although they may forget the way to the dining room. Carers should aim to provide support and help without taking over and encouraging the person to depend on staff for care before this is required.

If the person enters the home suffering from mild confusion and the early stages of dementia, carers get to know the person. When the person deteriorates and is unable to communicate needs to carers this is seldom a problem because the carers know the person very well. If a person is admitted to the home with advanced dementia it can be difficult to provide the type of care the person would prefer because staff do not know the person. Relatives and friends can be a great help in these circumstances. They can tell staff what food the person prefers, what her interests are, how she likes to dress and style her hair. In some homes a written record of this is kept so that all staff can treat the person as he or she would wish.

Communicating with confused patients

Some staff think that if an older person is confused and mistakes the time of day or a person, carers should 'play along' with this. Research over the last 40 years has shown that carers can do a great deal to lessen the older person's degree of confusion and to help the person to cope with memory loss. If the carer enters the room and the person says, 'Ah, it's Mary, isn't it, come to give me my lunch . . .', the carer should reply truthfully, 'No Mrs Anderson, it's Julie. It's breakfast time and I've brought breakfast. It's very bright in the morning in the summer isn't it. June is my favourite month.' The carer has reminded the person of her name and the time of day. She has also reminded her of the month.

Golden rules to help communication with confused patients

- carers should stick to the point and only talk about one thing at a time – people with dementia can only concentrate for short periods and a long conversation about several subjects can be difficult for them to follow
- do not give too much information at once
- break up a conversation or instructions into a series of small steps
- check that the person has understood
- repeat the information in a slightly different way
- be aware that the next day you may have to go through exactly the same routine again as the person may have forgotten
- listen to the older person
- check that you have understood what they are saying
- use touch and gestures to help communicate

Further information on communication is given in Chapter 2.

Wandering

Some older people wander around the home. This wandering can upset other patients and can make staff feel on edge. Although the older person appears to be wandering around aimlessly, they have a reason for wandering. Unfortunately not all people suffering from dementia wander for the same reasons. Research has shown that people who wander have great difficulty in communicating their needs. It has been suggested that the person's wandering is an attempt to meet those needs. If staff are able to identify and meet the person's needs then the person no longer wanders because the reason for wandering no longer exists. Causes of wandering may include:

- pain – the patient's facial expression, gestures and movements can indicate pain
- looking for the toilet – the person may not be able to remember where it is and all the doors look the same
- constipation – may be causing discomfort

- hunger – are the portions of food sufficient for an active person; are snacks available
- thirst – are drinks available
- is it too noisy – the person may want to find somewhere quiet and peaceful
- boredom – does the person want something to do
- is the person looking for something – perhaps a book or a bag which has been lost or left in her room.

Shouting and screaming

Carers will meet patients who shout, scream or sing continually. Carers and other patients can find this behaviour difficult to cope with. A great deal can be done to help people who behave like this. Carers should ask a nurse or doctor to see the person. In many cases the person's GP will ask a nurse specialising in psychiatric nursing to see the person. The aim of treatment is first to discover the reasons for the person behaving in this way, and then to plan care to eliminate or reduce such behaviour.

Aggression

Some older people lash out and shout at, hit, kick and bite carers. In many cases the person is confused and may be unaware of the carer's intentions. Carers should do everything possible to ensure that the older person is aware of what is about to happen, for example: 'Mrs Greenslade, I'd like to help you to have a bath now.'

If the person understands what the carer's intentions are and what is happening, aggression is less likely to occur. If the person refuses to bathe, dress or get up, carers must not try to force them. This is unlawful and can lead to aggression. Try leaving the person and returning a little later. If the incident takes place in a residential home, carers should record details of the aggressive incident. In nursing homes carers should ensure that the registered nurse in charge is aware and that incidents are recorded.

If a person is aggressive the reasons for the aggression should be determined and care planned to avoid such incidents. Sometimes the older person is extremely aggressive and could injure staff or other patients when lashing out. Patients and staff should not be placed in this situation. If the person is very disturbed, he or she will require care from registered nurses specially trained in caring for people with mental health problems. These nurses are known as Registered Mental Nurses (RMN). This specialist care may be given either in hospital or more usually in a specialist nursing home known as an Elderly Mentally Infirm (EMI) home.

Conclusion

Caring for older people who are confused, who appear to wander aimlessly, who scream, shout or sing, can be difficult and frustrating. The way that staff handle patients who suffer from dementia influences that person's behaviour. Staff attitudes and care can reduce or increase problems. Carers may see staff treat people with dementia as if they are children. Carers may be told, 'They're just babies really'.

Older people with dementia are not babies and are not 'in their second childhood', but are older people suffering from an incurable disease which affects brain function. Treating such people as babies not only denies them the dignity and respect which they deserve, but also worsens problem behaviour and increases the likelihood of abuse.

The likelihood of abuse is increased because staff can come to view patients as less than human. People with dementia can be seen not as people suffering from a dreadful incurable disease, but as objects. Carers who provide thoughtful sensitive care and ensure that the older person is treated with dignity and respect will find the older person responds to such care and that problem behaviour is very rare. Reading and attending study days will help the carer gain further knowledge about how to provide such care.

Portfolio preparation

Some NVQ students worry about this module and feel that if they have not actually witnessed or dealt with abuse, the module cannot be completed. The aim of the module is to raise awareness of abuse, of how to work in ways which minimize the risk of abuse, and of the range of actions which can be taken if abuse occurs. The following activities may help you to prepare your portfolio:

- Collect copies of any policies relating to abuse within your home.
- Give details of training available to help staff care for confused patients.
- Outline ways in which you think care within the home is organized and how this will reduce or increase the likelihood of abuse.
- Collect information from the organizations listed below and use this as part of your portfolio information.

Further information

Alzheimer's Disease Society
Gordon House
10 Greencoat Place
London SW1P 1PH.
Telephone 0171 306 0606

This society provides information and advice to relatives and staff who care for people with dementia. They produce a range of free fact sheets, books and a monthly newsletter. They run a series of courses for carers who work with older people suffering from dementia.

National organizations who provide advice and information

Action on Elder Abuse
Astral House
1268 London Road
London SW16 4ER.
Telephone 0181 679 2648

This charity provides information and leaflets including: *Elder Abuse in Care Homes* and *Abuse of Elderly People: Guidelines for Action.* These are available free of charge (send an SAE).

Age Concern (England)
Astral House
1268 London Road
London SW16 4ER.
Telephone 0171 679 8000

Age Concern offer information and advice on nursing and residential home care. They produce a range of leaflets, fact sheets and information.

Counsel and Care
Twyman House
16 Bonny Street
London NW1 9PG.
Telephone 0171 485 1566

Counsel and Care offer information and advice on nursing and residential home care. They have published a number of books, and have an advice line.

Public Concern at Work
Lincoln's Inn House
42 Kingsway
London WC2B 6EN.
Telephone 0171 404 6609

Public Concern at Work is a legal advice centre. They offer information and support.

Further reading

Hicks, C. (1988) *Who Cares. Looking After Older People at Home.* Virago Press, London.

Tomlin, S. (1988) *Abuse of Elderly People: An Unnecessary Problem.* Public information report. British Geriatrics Society, London.

Eastman, M. (1995) (Ed.) *Old Age Abuse: A New Perspective.* Age Concern and Chapman Hall (co-publishers), London.

Harvey, M. (1990) *Who's confused?* Prepar Publications, Birmingham.

Stokes, G. (1988) *Wandering.* Winslow Press, Bicester.

Stokes, G. (1988) *Screaming and Shouting.* Winslow Press, Bicester.

Chapter 4

Supporting Older People and Their Families

Introduction

This chapter gives information on:

- Living at home
- Life in a home
- Enabling older people to retain their identities
- Living life to the full
- The benefits of activities and interests
- Activities and interests
- How families feel about homes
- How staff view families
- Helping, supporting and welcoming families
- Enabling older people to see visitors in private

Life at home

Most older people live independent lives and do not require care. The people who enter homes are the most frail and ill of their generation. It is easy for us to lose sight of this when working in homes and to assume that all 85-year-old women have difficulty in caring for themselves. It is also easy for us to forget that the person who has come to the home may until recently have been living a full and independent life in their own home, where they could live life as they wished.

Doris Smith is a widow who has lived alone for five years. She decides what time to get up, what to eat for breakfast, when to wash, what to eat for lunch, what to do during the day. She decides to listen to the radio, or read a book or watch television.

Entering a home

Suddenly Mrs Smith's life is shattered. She suffers a stroke. A few weeks after the stroke she is visited by her family and the care manager who inform her that she will not be able to manage at home any more. A home is suggested. Mrs Smith is informed that she needs long-term care. This will mean having to give up her home, clear the house full of memories and the possessions of a lifetime and enter a home.

Suddenly Mrs Smith, who has always valued her independence and declined offers to move in with her daughter, is no longer in control. The home she enters is clean and tidy but she cannot bring her own furniture. The home has a routine and because Mrs Smith has difficulty in communicating the staff do not realise that she is alert. Mrs Smith is 'got up' when it is convenient for the staff. Breakfast is at 8AM and no one asks Mrs Smith if she would prefer to eat earlier or later. Mrs Smith has some difficulty in swallowing because of the stroke, so she has porridge, tea, white bread and butter and marmalade for breakfast. Mrs Smith would love a lightly poached egg on brown bread and a cup of black coffee.

Mrs Smith is bathed twice a week on Sundays and Wednesdays and is bedbathed on all other days. She prefers to shower each day. Mrs Smith's daughter has brought her clothes in from home. Her wardrobe, like every other woman's, contains clothes she rarely wears because she has 'gone off' them. Now no one asks her what she likes to wear and she is often dressed in that red dress she kept meaning to throw out. Mrs Smith is not able to make any real choices about her life. She is dependent on the staff at the home to help her. If she is sat next to someone with whom she has little in common she cannot go and sit elsewhere.

Enabling older people to retain their identities

Mrs Smith's fictional experience may seem far fetched but it shows how easy it is for people to lose their identities just because they are old and sick. Mrs Smith has entered the home at her lowest ebb. Staff who realise this, get to know her as a person and take time to discover her needs and wishes will make a real difference to her quality of life.

Mrs Smith would benefit from a full assessment by a speech and language therapist who could advise staff of the best ways to help Mrs Smith communicate. In the meantime staff could take time to find out Mrs Smith's wishes – further details are given in Chapter 2. Mrs Smith's daughter could help and advise staff. She would be able to tell them that Mrs Smith prefers black coffee, has never liked that red dress and would feel much better if her hair was cut and permed in her normal style. Mrs Smith and the staff could begin to form a relationship and work together to help her regain as much independence as possible.

Seeing someone like Mrs Smith enter a home feeling that it is the end of the world, and having the opportunity to work with her and see her improve mentally and physically, is so rewarding. It is, after all, the reason we all decided to work with older people.

Living life to the full

Often when we ask people what they do for a living we learn a lot about them. In some homes staff do not know very much about the older person's life. Is Mr Robinson a retired school teacher or a mechanic? If we are to help older people to retain their identities when living in homes, we need to know who they are. What is the older person's background? What interests has that person followed throughout life? In some homes staff keep a book and enter details of the person's life, interests, likes and dislikes. This can help all staff not only to see the whole person but also to give care that the person wants.

Mrs Anderson for example is a retired music teacher. Her eyesight is fading but she enjoys listening to music on the radio or television. Julie Carson, a carer at the home, checks the radio and television programmes each week and marks any which she feels will interest Mrs Anderson. Julie then discusses these with Mrs Anderson and when Mrs Anderson has decided which she would like to hear, a note of them is made. Staff help Mrs Anderson to sit comfortably in her room and make sure that the radio or television is on the right channel for her to enjoy her concert.

Mrs Anderson dislikes Brussels sprouts, gravy, semolina and too much custard on her puddings. A note of her likes and dislikes has been made. Mrs Anderson has been able to retain her identity and is treated as an individual. This is good for her morale. It makes her feel cared for and valued. We all feel so much better when we are treated as individuals, and older people are no different to you and I.

Benefit of activities and interests

Homes are for living in and activities and interests make life worthwhile and interesting for many people. Activities have been shown to improve concentration and reduce boredom. Taking part in activities helps people to live full lives and this improves physical and mental wellbeing.

In the early 1980s many older people requiring long-term care were cared for in NHS units. These units were usually in geriatric hospitals built many years before. Older people were nursed in wards. There was little privacy and they were dressed in clothes supplied by the hospital laundry rather than in their own clothes. In many hospitals older people were not treated as individuals and there were few opportunities for them to pursue their interests.

It was thought that older people would enjoy a better quality of life if they were cared for in nursing homes. Four experimental nursing homes were set up and people were asked if they wished to move from the hospital to the nursing home. The homes aimed to provide care in an environment that was more like the older person's home than a hospital. Individuals had their own rooms, wore their own clothes and were encouraged to take part in activities and pursue their own interests.

The results were dramatic; people who had lived in the hospital for years began to take an interest in life again and their physical and mental health improved. Activities encourage older people to move around, to sit up, to concentrate and to take an interest in life. People who are more alert and involved are less likely to spend half of the day dozing in the chair and will normally sleep well at night without sleeping tablets.

Encouraging individual activities and interests

People come from many different backgrounds and they have different skills, interests, experiences and personalities. Older people who live in homes differ in their interests just as much as any other group of people. The activities offered in the home should take account of the different interests and personalities of the people living there. Some people are naturally chatty and outgoing and love company. Some patients rush to get ready and get to the lounge for coffee and a chat. Others are quieter and prefer to spend their days quietly away from the bustle and activity of others. In some homes patients are placed under some pressure by well-meaning staff to join in activities which have been organized.

If a person does not wish to take part in an activity the carer should ask why; some people long to join in but lack confidence. Carers can help support and encourage patients who lack confidence, to take part in activities. Some older people are embarrassed by their disabilities or worry that because of illness it will be difficult to participate. Carers can help by encouraging and offering practical help in such situations. Activities in the home should be organized to take account of disabilities and to enable individuals to participate. Some older people prefer their own company or that of their family and friends who visit. If the individual prefers not to take part in activities carers should respect the individual's wishes.

Organizing activities

Many larger homes employ an activities organiser. This person works with staff and patients to organize and co-ordinate activities within the home. Many people, when they think of activities, imagine a large group of people all doing the same thing. Well-organized activity programmes involve working with small groups of people and with individuals as well as large groups. At some homes a number of people come to the home for a few sessions each week. Activity sessions from different people offer a variety of activities.

In smaller homes staff are required to work with patients to organize activities. In this situation staff have to ensure that activities are not squeezed out by the other work in the home. Homes are busy places and there is always something to do. Activities are important and helping patients to pursue their interests and activities is a very important part of working in homes. Ask any older person what mattered most to them, the person who tidied the lockers or the one who found time to help patients begin a game of Scrabble.

Types of activities

Carers involved in activity programmes should aim to offer as wide a range of activities as possible. It is easy for people to become bored if only a limited range of activities is offered.

Games

Games are popular with many patients. Some older people have poor eyesight even with spectacles. Playing cards which are twice the normal size can be seen by people with poor eyesight. A large print version of Scrabble is available. People with poor eyesight can see this more easily and people suffering from diseases such as motor neurone disease, multiple sclerosis and arthritis will find them easier to handle.

Large easy-to-handle draughts are also available. Bingo is popular in many homes. Large print bingo cards are available. Many homes have radios or music centres which have micro-phones. The microphone can be used to call numbers so that patients who do not have perfect hearing can join in.

Music

Many people enjoy music. It is easy to build up a record collection for the home. A notice on the home's notice board and a letter to the local newspaper asking for records usually works well. If you ask what type of music people prefer you will normally find this varies from classical to popular music of the 1920s, 1930s and 1940s. In some homes popular music is played during the morning and classical in the evening.

Most local hospitals have hospital radio stations, and many of these also offer a tape service. A member of the radio team visits the home and speaks to a group of patients asking what type of music they prefer. The music is then taped and sent to the home. Tapes are usually exchanged twice weekly. Individual patients can also have a personal selection of music taped and sent to them regularly. This can be listened to in private or shared with other patients.

Sing-songs can also be popular. Tapes or records of favourite songs from musicals such as South Pacific can be bought. It is often possible to buy large print song books which help people join in. If song books are not available, the words can be typed out and printed in large print by someone with access to a computer. Carers can help by encouraging patients to join in and by joining in themselves.

Many homes have pianos which are seldom used because no one can play. Often a notice saying 'Volunteer wanted to play the piano for one hour a week' will bring offers flooding in. An advertisement in a newsagent's window costs very little, so it may be worth advertising. The local secondary school may have pupils who would enjoy playing.

Concerts

Concerts can be formal and involve the use of professional entertainers, but this can be expensive and your home may not be able to afford many such concerts. Local choirs, operatic societies and other groups may be willing to perform in the home. Details of local groups can be obtained from your local library or Citizens' Advice Bureau.

Arts and crafts

Painting and drawing are relaxing activities. Many people who are no longer able to take part in more active pursuits enjoy creating drawings, pictures, prints and collages. Some older people are talented artists and create impressive paintings, whilst others enjoy making birthday cards, Christmas cards and prints. Paper, pencils, pens, felt-tip pens and poster paints are inexpensive and give hours of pleasure (Fig. 4.1). When people have worked hard to produce work it can be admired and displayed in the person's room or in the lounge, dining room and hall.

Many women enjoy knitting. Some, though able to knit beautifully, find that it is difficult to read a pattern because the print is too small. They could use a magnifier, or large print knitting

Fig. 4.1 A patient colouring – not all activities are group activities.

patterns are available from: Carter & Parker Ltd, Gordon Mills, Guiseley, Leeds LS20 9PD. Patients who have poor eyesight who are still able to knit may have difficulty sewing up garments. Often another patient who enjoys sewing may be able to help finish off garments. Both may enjoy working together.

Pets
Most people who enter homes lived alone before entering the home. This may be because they never married or because they were widowed. Many people who live alone enjoy the companionship of pets. People who live alone and who have pets enjoy better health than those without pets. Stroking a cat or patting a dog has been shown to reduce blood pressure and help people to relax.

Some homes have a policy of allowing the older person with a pet to bring the pet to live at the home wherever possible. This is not always possible, however, as some breeds of dog require a lot of exercise and the older person who enters a home will rarely be able to take a dog for long walks. Many older people recognize these difficulties and ask a friend or relative to care for their dog when they enter a home. Most homes now encourage family and friends to bring the older person's dog to visit. Many other patients also enjoy such visits. Cats require less looking after and in some homes the older person may bring her cat to stay.

Grace Andrews was admitted to a nursing home after suffering from a severe stroke. She recovered well from the stroke and regained speech and mobility but remained quiet and withdrawn. Staff at the home discovered that when Mrs Andrews was in hospital her cat had been run over and killed. Mrs Andrews missed the companionship dreadfully. The local Cat's Protection League visited and Mrs Andrews 'adopted' a cat. Having the companionship of a cat made Mrs Andrews feel that life was worth living again (Fig. 4.2).

Fig. 4.2   Grace and her cat.

Some people have budgies as pets and most homes allow people to bring these with them when they enter the home.

Sport
Many older people enjoy watching sport. Football, boxing, tennis, horse racing and cricket are often shown on television. If the individual enjoys watching these carers can help by checking the

times of particular events and helping the person to enjoy them uninterrupted. The person who enjoys tennis should have chiropody treatment planned so that it will not coincide with matches at Wimbledon.

Many people enjoy watching sports events out of doors. If Mr Walters played rugby as a younger man he may enjoy watching a local rugby team. The team can be contacted and arrangements made for him to watch local matches. Many sports teams are extremely helpful and will help transport sports enthusiasts to their games and involve them in the social activities of the team. Sitting under a tree watching a cricket match or sitting in a pub watching the darts team play is a world away from how most people view homes. Carers can, with a little imagination and planning, help older people live life to the full within homes.

Exercise sessions

Exercise is not only for the young and fit. People of all ages can benefit from exercise; even frail and disabled people can take part. EXTEND (Exercise Training For the Elderly) is a charity which specialises in working with older people. Using music and a series of exercises which exercise different parts of the body, EXTEND aims to make people living in homes feel as well as possible.

Reading

Homes obtain books from the mobile library service which is run by the local council. Councils deliver a selection of books to homes and hospitals, and these are exchanged every few months. The library service ask the home which types of books are required. Most older people find it easier to read large print and there is now a large selection of large print books available. If an older person is an avid reader the library service can deliver a book (or two) to the individual. The library asks the person to fill in a form (usually large print) asking them their reading preferences and delivers and collects books on request. Some older people may prefer to go to the library and select their own books. Carers can escort and help patients who wish to do this.

Books for the blind and partially sighted

People who have very poor vision can be registered blind. The patient's doctor fills in a form and the person is registered with the local council. People who are registered blind or partially sighted are issued with special library tickets which enable them to take out tapes or books free of charge.

There are two sizes of book tape. The 'Talking Book' cassette recorders take larger cassettes. Talking Book cassettes are sent out in the post to registered blind people from a central library run by the council. The book cassettes available in local libraries fit into normal cassette players.

Television and films

Many older people enjoy watching television. It is important though that television is not seen as the only activity. In some homes the television is on all day and no one is listening. Carers can try to find out which television programmes patients like and let them know when these are on.

Many people like watching films, especially old films. If the home has a video recorder films can be taped and film shows organized in the evening. This can be made into an event, with drinks and popcorn available.

Homes – the family's view

Many older people are cared for at home before they enter homes. Others are living independent lives before an illness such as a stroke leads to hospital admission. The average older person living in a home is 85 years old. The older person's children are often retired and in their sixties and seventies. Many families feel that they have 'failed' when an older person is admitted to a home. Some families feel guilty that they could not care for the older person at home. Most older people who are admitted to homes require high levels of care and in most cases it would be impossible to provide this level of care at home, especially on a long-term basis. Some older people do not realise how much care they require and constantly ask their families to take them home. There have been a number of television programmes recently high-lighting poor care in homes. Many relatives are anxious about the care the home will offer; they worry about their loved one receiving the care and attention required.

Some relatives have struggled alone and without help or the specialist equipment that the home has, until they reach the end of their tether. The older person is admitted to the home and if care appears good the relative can feel inadequate, perhaps thinking 'Look how well the staff cope, yet I couldn't even look after my own mother'. In other cases the relative may be very critical of the care in the home and may think, 'What have I done putting her into a home?'

People who suffer from senile dementia gradually lose the ability to remember. In the end stages of the disease the older person no longer recognizes herself in the mirror and is often unable to recognize her family. A daughter who visits her mother in the home to find that her mother no longer recognizes her can become terribly upset by this.

The staff view

Carers sometimes feel that they cannot win with relatives. If the older person looks and feels well the relative feels guilty; if the older person appears unsettled and asks to go home the staff are not providing good care. Some relatives visit daily and appear to ask for information about every little detail of the patient's day. Others visit rarely and appear to take no interest in the patient.

Helping and supporting families

The older person's family want the best possible care for their loved one. Carers want to care for older people and to give the best possible care. Families and staff who work together as a team can make sure that the care the older person receives is of the best possible standard. It is important that carers take the time to get to know the older person's family and build up a good relationship. When the older person enters a home the family may be anxious and upset. The carer who understands the reasons why families feel this way will be able to build a relationship with the family. Families often feel that they can no longer have any say in the older person's life because they have 'handed over' to the staff at the home.

Relatives have known their loved one for a lifetime and know much more about the person than the staff do. If carers ask relatives for their help and advice, relatives will feel that they can continue to have some influence over the older person's life. The carer who chats to a relative might say, 'Yes, it is lovely today. I was going to ask if Mrs Harrison would like me to bring her to the shops in her wheelchair later. Do you think she'd like that?' The skilled carer can discuss how Mrs Harrison enjoys her trips to the shops when her daughter next visits. Within a few weeks Mrs Harrison's daughter may be taking her mother to the shops when she visits.

Relatives who cared for their loved one at home may feel failures when the older person enters a home. The carer who asks the relative for advice immediately builds a bond with the relative; for example the carer might ask:

'I noticed that Mrs Kay's skin is very dry. Has she had this problem before?'.

'Yes. I tried lots of creams but they weren't much good. In the end the doctor prescribed a cream which worked well. Would you like me to get the name of it for you. I think I've got it in my bag.'

When a relative has cared for a loved one at home the older person often becomes the centre of the relative's life. The relative may have dropped outside interests and lost touch with friends because all free time was devoted to caring. In such circumstances the relatives may be relieved that the loved one is happy and well cared for in a home. The relative may, however, feel guilty and may ask carers to assure her that she has done the right thing:

'You must think I'm wicked.'

'I do feel terrible about Mum being here, but she seems very happy.'

The carer might reply:

'She is happy but she does need a lot of care. It's easier for us here. We go home at night and the night staff take over. You did really well to care for her so well at home for such a long time.'

The carer is letting the relative know that the staff are not judging her and that they realise that caring for a loved one at home is not always possible.

In most areas the local council appoints a carers support co-ordinator. There are usually a number of local carers support groups, who meet regularly. Some members are carers and others are people who have a family member in a home. Relatives attending these groups can talk to other people in similar situations. The groups also organize social activities and this gives relatives the opportunity to meet others socially. The carers support co-ordinator can supply details of local groups. If your home does not have a contact number this can be obtained from the Citizen's Advice Bureau or the social services department in your town hall.

Helping families to remain involved

Many relatives are keen to remain involved in caring for their loved one. Some do not offer because they worry about offending staff. Other relatives have seen their loved one change from a healthy independent person to a disabled person. This change can literally happen overnight.

Mr Charles Webster was widowed some years ago. He remained active and did all his own shopping, cooking, cleaning and ironing. He visited his local pub twice a week and met his friends. One winter's evening he slipped over on the pavement on his way to the pub. He fell heavily and broke his leg. Surgeons at the local hospital operated but unfortunately Mr Webster suffered a heart attack. He was discharged to a home, unable to walk or care for himself.

Mr Webster gradually learnt to walk again and became more

independent. He was unable to walk long distances because of his heart condition. His son often visited the home and staff noticed that both father and son ran out of conversation after a few minutes. Both looked awkward.

One of the care assistants, Lily McDonald, asked how they normally spent their time together before Mr Webster's illness. She learnt that father and son normally went to the pub and had a chat over a pint. Lily suggested that they go to the pub during visits and offered to fetch a wheelchair so that the son could push his father to the pub. The son was frightened by the suggestion and thought that because his father had been ill he could not go out without a member of staff; it was too dangerous, anything might happen. He agreed to take his father to the pub if a member of staff accompanied them 'just in case'. After a few visits both father and son felt confident to go to the pub unaccompanied – much to the disappointment of staff!

Some relatives are equally worried about having a loved one home to tea. Carers can help by encouraging relatives and by accompanying the patient home for a trial visit. This can help patient and relative feel more confident.

Relatives can often help and encourage patients with exercises and therapy; for example, if an older person has speech difficulties after a stroke, staff can involve caring relatives in therapy.

Mrs Winifred Pearson was admitted to a home from hospital following a stroke. She was unable to speak. She was visited by a speech and language therapist who carried out an assessment and worked out a plan of care. Mrs Pearson's family took a day off work and met the speech and language therapist at the home. They worked with the staff at the home to help Mrs Pearson regain her speech.

Visiting

Visiting times

The home is now the older person's home. In their own home the older person would welcome friends and relatives. It is important that the home encourages the older person's family and friends to visit, and makes them feel welcome. Hospitals have visiting hours, and restricting visiting to certain hours helps ensure that hospital patients get enough rest and that treatment can be carried out. Hospital visiting hours are now more flexible than before and are normally from 2PM until 8PM.

Many homes do not have set visiting hours and welcome people throughout the day. Find out what the policy on visiting hours is in your home. Homes aim to provide care in a setting which is as normal and homelike as possible. At home people call when they are passing and when they have time. If the home has rigid visiting hours this can make it difficult for some people to visit and can put others off.

Some home managers fear that if there are no set visiting hours, the home will be over-run with visitors and it will be difficult to care for patients. This is not the case. An open visiting policy encourages people to visit and is probably less disruptive than a rush of visitors at 2PM on Sunday afternoons. Family, friends and neighbours can pop in and do not expect the home to look perfect at all times. If a doctor or therapist has arrived, visitors will leave if required and can return later.

Many older people look forward to visits from old friends of their own age group. If visiting hours start at 2PM and the visitor stays a few hours he or she may have to travel home in the dark on a winter's evening. The prospect of this can put some older people off visiting and can deprive patients of the company of their dearest friends.

Some relatives work and if visiting ends at 8PM, for example, the relative may have to rush straight from work to the home. The relative may be tired and hungry and may only visit for a short time. Sometimes the relative may decide not to visit. If relatives can visit later in the evening there is time to go home, eat and relax before the visit. The relative will be encouraged to visit more often and stay longer.

Many older people in homes look forward to visits but too many visitors at once can be tiring; an open visiting policy enables people to spread their visits through the day. The older person has an opportunity to chat at length with each visitor. Some older people go to bed early in the evening because they are bored and have nothing to look forward to. An evening visit brightens the evening and prevents boredom.

Welcoming visitors

Many visitors travel long distances to visit the home; others have come direct from work. It is normal to offer visitors refreshments when they visit our own homes, and offering visitors a cup of tea or coffee makes them feel welcome. At times the home may be busy and it can be difficult to find time to make tea. Perhaps your home could offer tea and coffee making facilities so that visitors can help themselves in such circumstances.

Privacy during visits

Some older people have difficulty hearing. They may not enjoy a visit if they have to strain to hear above background noise in a lounge. Everyone has the right to privacy during visits. Some people prefer to remain in a communal area, such as a lounge, while others prefer to see their visitors in the privacy of their room. Some older people have difficulty in walking and require assistance to get to and from their rooms. Carers should be sensitive to the needs of visitors and patients and should offer to assist patients to their rooms if they wish to enjoy a visit in private.

Visitors can be encouraged to take the older person out on short trips to the shops, to the local café or to the park if they wish. All 'visits' do not have to take place within the home. Check how your home encourages and involves visitors.

Summary

Older people living in their own home make decisions about their lives. They are free to pursue their own interests and to welcome family, friends and neighbours into their homes. Staff should aim to enable older people living in homes to live as full a life as possible within the home. Each person is unique and has their own personality and interests; carers should work with older people and their families to help people retain their interests.

Families often worry and feel guilty when a loved one enters a home; they want only the best for their loved one. The relationship carers build up with the older person's friends and family is just as important as the one between carers and patients. Carers can work with families to provide the best possible care for older people.

Portfolio preparation

- Draw up a list of ways in which staff in your home work to enable older people to retain their identities.
- If your home has a formal activities programme make a copy of it and include it in your portfolio.
- Chat to an older person in the home and ask about how life at home differed from life in the home. Include this information in your portfolio.
- List ways that families are involved in the care of the people in the home.

Chapter 5

Support when Moving to a New Environment

Introduction

This chapter gives information which will enable the carer to support the older person who moves into a new environment. The chapter includes:

- why older people need support
- preparing for admission
- admission to the home
- supporting the older person on admission
- dignity and privacy in homes
- hospital admissions, emergency and planned
- day surgery
- outpatients visits
- rehabilitation
- respite care

Why older people need support

Few of us have any idea of how distressing and worrying it is to enter a home. For us the home is our place of work and it holds no terrors for us. If we are unhappy in the home we can always leave. Most older people are admitted to homes from hospital. In most cases the admission to hospital was because of a sudden illness or accident. In other cases the older person may have been admitted to hospital because an existing condition, such as arthritis or Parkinson's disease, became much worse. When people go to hospital they expect to have an operation or treatment, get better and go home. It can be a terrible shock for the older person to be told that she must leave hospital but cannot go home.

Most older people given a choice would avoid homes and would prefer to return to their own homes. People entering homes may have moved from their own home to hospital, had treatment and may have been moved to another ward before entering the home. The individual may dread the thought of another move and may worry about the staff. Will they be friendly and kind? Will I get the help I need? What is it going to be like?

Carers should be aware of the fears and anxieties people will experience when entering a home. A little time and trouble taken in getting to know the individual and offering support will help allay the person's fears.

Preparing for admission

In many homes patients are encouraged to bring items from home to make their room seem like home. Many older people have framed photographs of their families which they treasure. The individual's family can bring in framed photographs and pictures from home and these can be hung on hooks on walls. Ornaments brought from home can be placed around the room. The individual may have a favourite chair, cushions and footstool. These could be placed in the room. Some individuals may wish to bring in other items of furniture such as small tables, a bed, wardrobe, china cabinet or bureau. If the individual can bring treasured items to the home, it becomes more like moving home than being 'put in a home'. Some individuals may wish to bring bedspreads or bed-covers from home.

Most homes have fully furnished rooms but there is no reason why this furniture cannot be stored so that the individual can bring in her own belongings. Older people who become involved in planning the move to a home, and who can decide which items to bring with them, normally feel more positive about entering the home. Some homes do not allow people to bring in furniture and bedding because they fear that the fire officer will not allow this. In homes mattresses and all soft furnishings have to meet specific fire retardancy standards. These regulations and guidelines were introduced to make homes as safe as possible. They were not, however, introduced to prevent elderly people from bringing treasured items from home. Most fire officers, if asked about this, state that the home *must* purchase items which meet fire retardancy standards and that individuals may bring items from home which do not meet these standards.

Carers should make sure that the room is prepared for the person's arrival. Make sure fresh water and a glass are supplied. Check that the bed is made neatly and there are towels available. If the room appears stuffy air it, remembering to close the window a few hours before the person is expected, if it is cold outside. If it is cold check that the heating is on. Make sure that the lights and the call bell work; if not, arrange repairs quickly. Check that the wardrobe has hangers in it and that the drawers and locker are clean. If possible place a flowering plant or some flowers in the room. The older person will find that the room is warm, comfortable and welcoming when she arrives.

Admission to the home

Most older people are admitted to homes from hospitals and are transferred to the home by ambulance. The individual may have waited either on the ward or in the hospital transport department for many hours before commencing the journey to the home. In some ambulances a number of people are transported at once so the journey may take some time. By the time the older person arrives at the home her bladder may be full to bursting, and she may be tired, hungry, thirsty or in pain. Carers should be sensitive to these possibilities; now is not the time to introduce her to all the other residents or launch into lengthy admission procedures. Introducing yourself and helping the person to her room is best. When the person's immediate needs have been met the admission procedures can begin. If the person is very tired she may wish to rest for a few hours first.

On first name terms?

These days people often use first names even when addressing people they do not know well. The people admitted to homes come from a different generation. They were, in their youth, addressed by their title and surname in many situations and first names were used only by close friends and family. Some older people view the way we use first names now as refreshing and friendly; others may think it over-familiar or patronising. We address children by their first names but use titles and surnames as a mark of respect. It is important to ask the individual how he or she wishes to be addressed and to use that form of address. The person who wishes to be addressed as Mrs Harley-Smith may in time ask her carers to call her Ellen. Some older people, like younger people, dislike their names and use a nickname or a completely different first name. Mrs Dorothy Mason for example may be called Anne by her friends. The carer should make a note in the care plan or inform senior staff of how the person prefers to be addressed.

Supporting the individual after admission

People entering the home normally require a lot of help and support in the first month of admission. It takes time for the person to settle in and discover how the home is run. The aim of care in homes is for care to be centred around the patient. The patient, though, will need a little time and some guidance to develop a routine which suits his or her needs. Most people develop routines in their lives and people living in homes are no different. A routine offers structure to the day but should be flexible enough to enable the individual to enjoy life.

The person entering the home has to learn a great deal: the names of the staff, mealtimes, visiting times, arrangements for laundry, when activities take place. If the individual is given too much information at once, it can be difficult for them to remember it all. It is also difficult to decide which information is the most important. To the keen reader the location of the library books is very important, whilst to another individual that is of minor interest.

Some homes now produce information books which provide a great deal of information about the home. These are usually made up of loose leaf sheets held in plastic sleeves in a ring binder. Information can be updated quickly and easily. The new patient can read through the information book and find the information which is important to him or her.

Dignity and privacy

One of the things many older people fear most on entering a home is the loss of dignity and privacy. At home the older person's privacy was protected by her front door; before anyone could enter she had to open it. In homes some rooms do not have locks. Disabilities may prevent the older person from locking her room door in other homes. Imagine what it must be like to have people barging into your room without knocking. In some homes room doors are not even closed and the older person can be seen by anyone walking along the corridor. Carers should always knock and ask permission before entering a person's room.

Some patients, especially those living in nursing homes, are more disabled than others. Some disabled people depend on carers to get clothing from wardrobes and chests of drawers. Carers should always ask the person's permission before getting clothing and items out.

Sharing rooms

In some homes patients do not have their own room but share the room with one or more people. Carers should be very careful to safeguard the person's privacy and dignity in such situations. The individual may have been living alone for many years and may be very embarrassed about sharing a room with others. In sharing rooms each bed has bedcurtains. These should be used to protect the person's privacy when she is washing, dressing, using a commode or bedpan, or wishes to have them drawn. If the room has a washbasin, this will also have curtains. These should be used to maintain the person's privacy when washing.

Hospital admission

People living in homes are more acutely ill than before and the number of people being re-admitted to hospital from homes has risen rapidly in the last two years. Older people living in residential homes are more likely to be re-admitted to hospitals than those living in nursing homes. There are three different types of admission: emergency admission, planned admission, and day surgery.

Emergency admissions

Emergency admissions are, of course, unplanned. The older person may have fallen and a fracture is suspected, or she may have become acutely ill and require hospital treatment. There is no time to prepare for the admission and the person who has settled into the home suddenly has to cope with the stress of returning to hospital. The individual is often worried about her health and the prospect of leaving the home and returning to hospital. If the person is very ill there is little time to prepare and often the carer only has time to prepare a toilet bag.

In emergency situations patients are taken to the accident and emergency department (A & E) where they are assessed and investigated and the doctors decide if the person requires hospital treatment. If the person's GP has arranged the emergency admission, the GP will write a letter to the medical staff in A & E. Sometimes the staff at the home have called for an ambulance and the patient has not been seen by a GP. In these circumstances the person in charge of the home will write a letter giving details of the person's medical history, the current problem and details of any medicines which the individual is taking.

It is good practice for staff from the home to escort any patient requiring emergency treatment to the hospital. In nursing homes if the person is seriously ill a registered nurse will accompany the patient, if staffing levels allow. In smaller homes and in residential homes carers may find themselves accompanying an acutely ill person to hospital. Each emergency ambulance is fully equipped and has two trained paramedical staff. Both are specially trained in caring for acutely ill people. The carer's role is to reassure and support the patient and to communicate with hospital staff on arrival at the hospital.

Hospital accident and emergency departments can be very busy. The carer should stay with the older person, accompany her to X-ray if required, explain procedures, and provide practical help and moral support. When the individual is admitted to the ward the carer should remain until the person is settled in. Find out as much as possible about the plan of treatment before leaving. If possible try to get some indication of how long the person is expected to remain in hospital. The individual's glasses, dentures, hearing aid and walking frame may have been left at the home.

It is estimated that 10% of all people living in homes have no close relatives or friends. While it is important to keep in touch with all patients who are in hospital, those without family or friends may feel particularly alone and lost. A daily telephone call to check how the individual is progressing, and to leave a message for them, will help the person feel she is not forgotten. If possible visit the person in hospital; telephone first to check if she requires anything from home. Visiting, bringing fresh clothes and a small gift such as a plant, magazine or some fruit, helps the carer remain in contact with the person.

Many older people worry that if they become ill or require greater levels of care than before, the home will refuse to have them back. Residential homes do not normally employ registered nurses and employ fewer staff than nursing homes. In some cases if the older person becomes more disabled she may be unable to return to the residential home. Some nursing homes care for older people who require high levels of skilled care, whilst others are unable to cope with this. It is important that the carer finds out what level of care is provided within the home. If an individual is worried that she will be unable to return to the home inform your manager who can visit, discuss this with the patient and in the vast majority of cases set the person's mind at rest.

People returning to the home after a hospital stay may be weaker and less able to care for themselves than previously. It may take time for the individual to regain strength and ability after an illness. The patient's room should be prepared ready for re-admission and any get well cards from friends, relatives, patients and staff put in the room.

Planned admissions

In the past older people in homes were seldom re-admitted to hospital for non-emergency treatment. Now, though, attitudes are more positive and medical staff are more aware that in some cases hospital treatment may improve an older person's quality of life. Planned hospital treatment is becoming more common.

When non-emergency treatment is required there is time to prepare and support the person. The carer should find out as much as possible about treatment planned. Normally hospital and professional staff working in homes explain the treatment in detail; however patients may wish to discuss the treatment with the carer. Carers should seek professional advice if they are unable to provide information required by individuals.

Day surgery

Day surgery is becoming very common. Now people who a few years ago would have remained in hospital for a few days after surgery are admitted in the morning and discharged home in the evening. It is possible to treat greater numbers of people on a day surgery basis. Many older people who develop cataracts find that instead of joining long waiting lists they can be treated quickly on a day surgery basis.

People requiring day surgery are normally sent by their GP to see a specialist at the local hospital. If the specialist feels that the surgery can be carried out as day surgery the person is placed on a waiting list. A short time before planned admission (usually a week) the patient visits the day surgery unit for assessment and investigation, and professional staff give full details of the planned surgery and the care required afterwards. Most surgery units supply written patient information booklets.

On the day of the operation, if a general anaesthetic is required the person does not eat or drink. (The day surgery unit will supply instructions about eating and drinking.) Many cases of day surgery are carried out under local anaesthetic. The person is normally admitted to the ward in the morning, prepared for surgery and taken to theatre. After the operation the patient usually rests for some time, nursing staff carry out routine post-operative checks and the doctor examines the patient before agreeing discharge if all is well.

It is policy in most homes that a member of staff accompanies the individual to the hospital and remains at the hospital providing support and practical help during the person's stay. If you are to escort a patient to day surgery and wish to watch the operation discuss this with your manager. The nurse in charge of the day surgery unit can ask the surgeon if you can enter the theatre and observe the operation. Many surgeons explain the operation as they carry it out.

Many older people become more and more worried about day

surgery as the day of the operation approaches. Knowing that a carer will remain at the hospital throughout the day reassures many older people.

Outpatient visits

Visits to the hospital outpatient department may be required for a number of reasons:

- following surgery at the hospital
- to check on an existing medical condition
- to consider if further treatment is required for a specific problem

In some homes all older people are escorted to outpatients appointments by a member of staff. In other homes transport is arranged to the hospital but the home does not provide an escort. In some cases a member of the patient's family arranges to meet her at the hospital. Almost all nursing homes provide escorts, whilst the policy in residential homes varies.

Carers who are asked to escort an older person to an outpatient's appointment should make sure that they know the purpose of the visit. Is it a routine check up? Is it to discuss possible further treatment? The patient should have an appointment card giving details of which clinic she is to attend, the doctor she is seeing and the time of the appointment. Senior staff may also send a letter giving details of current medication and treatment.

If ambulance transport has been arranged it is important to bear in mind that ambulances can arrive very much earlier or later than ordered. Help the person get ready in plenty of time. An early breakfast or lunch may be required. When transport arrives it may be picking up a number of other people before going to the hospital. Ask the individual if she wishes to use the toilet before leaving. If it is cold outside make sure the individual's coat is at hand and help her to put it on before leaving.

You may find that you have to wait a few hours in outpatients before the patient is seen, so be prepared. Take some 20p pieces so that you can both have a cup of tea while waiting; most outpatients departments have vending machines. Take extra change so that you can telephone the home if there is a problem getting transport back. Take something to pass the time; perhaps magazines, the patient's knitting or some playing cards. When the doctor sees the patient check that you both understand the outcome of the visit. On returning to the home the individual may be feeling tired after the journey. Be sensitive to her needs and offer the opportunity to rest if she wishes. Inform the person in charge of the outcome of the visit.

Rehabilitation

Greater numbers of old people are now admitted to homes so that they can fully recover from operation or illness and return home. If the individual is admitted to the home for a short stay the carer will normally work with a range of other staff to help prepare the person for discharge home. Many staff, such as the physiotherapist and occupational therapist, and the GP will be working with the older person to help her to regain the ability to care for herself at home. The carer's role is to work with others to ensure that every member of the team is working with the patient to the same aim. Recovering after a major illness is hard work, and there will be times when the older person feels low. The carer can offer encouragement and support at such times.

Respite care

There are seven million people caring for older people in their own homes in the UK. They care for relatives or friends who would otherwise require long-term care. For many years carers have not received the help required to enable them to continue to care. Now respite care is becoming more available and homes will be caring for more people on a respite basis in the next few years.

Respite care is a planned period of care. The older person is admitted to the home for a short period, normally two weeks on a regular basis, so that the carer can have a break. Caring for an older person at home without assistance is extremely demanding. Many carers find it difficult to do the things which we take for granted, such as go to the shops or visit friends. The aim of respite care is to enable carers to continue caring for longer periods by offering planned breaks.

In homes a number of beds are booked as respite beds. The individual is booked in for certain weeks throughout the year. Many older people who are admitted for respite care for the first time worry that they will never return home. Carers should be sensitive to such fears and reassure individuals that this is a temporary admission. Many carers have developed ways of meeting the older person's needs at home and have developed a routine. It is important that staff obtain as much information as possible about the older person's normal care and routine and do not disrupt this. It may be easier for two members of staff to help the person onto the toilet but if the carer and the older person live alone and have been managing, carers will only make life more difficult when the older person returns home. If the person's bedroom at home is upstairs staff should be careful to continue walking upstairs with the older person and not use the lift. If the older person loses the ability to walk upstairs, how will she cope at home?

During the period of respite care staff may be able to help organize services such as chiropody or suggest that aids such as grab rails may help the older person manage at home. Such suggestions and offers of help should be made sensitively as the carers may feel that staff are critical of their ability to cope. Many older people and their carers benefit from regular respite care and find that the support of staff in the early days is vitally important.

Summary

The role of homes is changing rapidly. Now older people move from hospital to home and home to hospital more than ever before. Change is difficult to cope with at the best of times, and older people who have been ill or who have undergone recent surgery can feel very vulnerable and worried as they move between care environments. Carers who are aware of older people's worries can respond sensitively and help individuals adjust to changing circumstances.

Portfolio preparation

- If your home has a brochure include this in your portfolio.
- Ask if you can photocopy policies which are aimed to support a person moving into the home.
- The home may have policies on assessment before admission, dignity and privacy. Ask if you can take copies and include these in your portfolio.
- Outline ways in which older people are welcomed and supported when they first enter the home.
- Find out the home's policy on escorting patients to outpatients appointments. Include copies of any written policies if possible.
- Find out if it is the policy for a member of staff to escort a patient to hospital if emergency treatment is required.
- What methods are used to keep in touch with patients when they are in hospital having treatment? Collect details for your portfolio.

Further reading

Alzheimer's Disease Society (1993) *Deprivation & Dementia*. A report by the Alzheimer's Disease Society, London. This report discusses the resources needed to help carers continue to provide care. It gives a series of case studies which illustrate the difficulties carers face when caring for a relative at home.

Carers National Association (1993) *Listening to Carers*. Carers National Association, London. This book discusses the services carers need to help them continue to care for relatives at home.

Chapter 6

Health and Safety Within the Home

Introduction

The aim of this chapter is to outline how carers can contribute to maintaining the health and safety not only of older people but also of visitors and colleagues within the home. The chapter includes information on:

- safety and security within the home
- who can enter the home
- the Health & Safety at Work Act – employer and employee responsibilities
- action to be taken in the event of fire
- what to do if a patient is missing
- recording details of patient's money
- caring for valuable and precious items
- preventing accidents
- recording and learning lessons from accidents
- identifying patients at risk of accidents
- balancing the risk of accident against the quality of life
- restraint
- medical emergencies.

Safety and security within the home

Health and safety is an important issue but one that does not always receive the attention it should. Most people do not like to think about accidents and tend to put thoughts about health and safety to the back of their minds. Accidents are less likely to occur if every member of staff is aware of how accidents can occur and works in ways which reduce the risk of accidents occurring. More details about this are given later in the chapter.

Older people living in homes and staff working within homes can be vulnerable to attack. There have been cases where intruders have entered homes and robbed and attacked staff and patients. In some cases staff and patients have been seriously injured. In the past many homes left the front entrance to the home 'on the latch' so that visitors could enter without having to be let in. Now the majority of homes have the front door closed and visitors must ring the doorbell. This increases the safety and security of the people in the home. Staff are also more aware of who is in the building and this is important if a fire occurs. Some homes still leave a side entrance open during daylight hours. At night it is the policy in most homes that doors are locked and ground floor windows (apart from fanlights) are closed. Check what policies your home has for ensuring security.

Who can enter the home

Nursing and residential homes are the homes of older people; they are not public places and there is no automatic right of entry for the public. In practice people who have a purpose in visiting the home, such as relatives and friends of patients and people who have come to deliver goods or services, are allowed free entry to the home. If a person living in the home does not wish to see someone (perhaps a neighbour), the neighbour has no right to enter the home.

Certain people have the legal right to enter the home. These are:

- registration officers
- employees of the electricity board who may wish to read the meter
- employees of the gas board who may wish to read the meter or investigate possible gas leaks
- employees of the water board who may wish to read the water meter (most homes now have water meters and are charged according to how much water is used) or investigate possible water leaks
- fire officers who are employed by the fire brigade and have the power to visit the home and check that fire precautions are satisfactory
- members of the local fire brigade who may wish to familiarise themselves with the layout of the home – this enables them to evacuate patients quickly and safely if required because of a fire
- health and safety officers employed to ensure that health and safety standards are met
- environmental health officers who ensure that food handling and storage is satisfactory and that policies on waste disposal are satisfactory
- pharmacists employed by the local NHS trust to ensure that medicines are stored and administered correctly

Although these groups of people have the legal right to enter the home, staff should check the person's identification before allowing entry.

Health and safety policy

Employers have certain duties under the Health and Safety Act 1974. The aim of the Act is to ensure that the employer takes care to ensure the health and safety of employees and also people living in or entering the home. Some of these duties are explained here.

Taking precautions to reduce accidents

This means that if an employer is aware of some problem which may cause an accident, steps should be taken to prevent accidents occurring. If the employer knows that a carpet is frayed and could cause some one to trip but takes no action, a breach of the Act has occurred. There have been cases where employers have been prosecuted for failing to clear snow from paths because accidents have occurred.

Employers who have more than five employees are required to have a policy statement

This details the employer's responsibilities and the staff's responsibilities. The policy statement may give details about special precautions to be taken to prevent accidents; for example, it may be policy for domestic staff to leave signs saying 'Caution wet floor' on floors which they have just mopped. The policy statement may also give detailed instructions about the safe-keeping of items such as cleaning materials and medicines. It will also instruct all employees about action they should take if they become aware of a hazard or a breach of the health and safety policy.

Employers are required to provide adequate training of staff to prevent accidents

In homes this will mean that staff who are required to move patients should have regular instruction and updating in lifting. Further details are given in Chapter 9.

Employers have a duty to provide equipment to prevent accidents

This means that employers should provide a range of equipment, from rubber gloves and overalls for domestics required to clean toilets, to hoists for staff required to move patients.

Employers have a duty to ensure that staff are aware of what action they must take during emergencies

The emergencies are:

- fire
- accident
- a missing patient.

Staff responsibilities under the Health & Safety Act

Staff working within the home have duties and responsibilities to work in ways that reduce the risk of accidents and make the home as safe as possible. Most of these are common sense.

Cleaning materials

Many cleaning materials are very toxic. Bleach and toilet cleaners can damage the skin and cause serious injury if drunk. Other cleaning materials may not appear dangerous but can cause accidents; for example, spilt washing-up liquid can cause a fall. In residential homes carers may be responsible for cleaning as well as caring. Carers should ensure that all cleaning materials are kept locked away. It may be convenient to have the toilet cleaner by the side of the toilet but this could cause serious harm to a confused patient.

Nursing homes normally employ domestic staff but the carer may find cleaning materials left out. The carer has a duty to remove these from patient areas to prevent the possibility of injury.

Medications

In nursing homes medicines are stored in a locked cabinet and only trained staff have access to the drugs cupboard or trolley. Medicines which are being returned to the pharmacy are often stored in the treatment room. Creams and lotions are also stored in the treatment room. Treatment rooms are locked. Carers should make sure they always lock treatment room doors after leaving. In residential homes some patients keep their own medicines and take them when prescribed. If the older person leaves her medicine lying around there is a danger that a confused patient might take these medicines. If the carer is worried about such a situation she should consult the home manager or a senior member of staff.

Fire training

Every person working in the home should be aware of what to do in case of fire. Each person working in the home should be given training in this and should attend a fire drill every six months. It is important that you are aware of where each fire exit is and what to do in case of fire.

Normally when the fire alarm goes off all staff report to a fire assembly point. Find out where the fire assembly point is in your home. It is usually by the main panel of the fire alarm. The fire alarm in homes normally has one large panel and a number of smaller panels. The home is divided into zones and the rooms and areas covered by each zone will be written on the fire panel; for example, zone one might be the lounge, kitchen and laundry. If a fire has occurred in zone one staff would check in which part of this area the fire had occurred. If the fire alarm has been triggered in the kitchen by burning toast the action taken would be different from that required if the deep fat fryer was in flames.

Find out if your home has written guidance on what action is to be taken in case of fire. Many homes have this guidance framed and hung on the wall next to fire alarm panels.

Fire exits

All fire exits in the home should be clearly marked and should be kept clear at all times. It is easy though for busy staff to allow fire exits to become blocked. A delivery of stationery or goods may be left blocking a fire exit as staff intend to put things away later. Relatives can easily place a chair in front of the fire exit in the lounge and then leave without putting it back. Homes are for living in but it is important that carers are aware that blocked exits cause delay in evacuating the home if a fire breaks out. At times carers must exercise great tact in ensuring that patients and their families are not offended, but that exits are kept clear.

Accident policy

The aim of all accident policies is to prevent accidents occurring whenever possible. It is not possible to make any home completely safe and this will be discussed later in the chapter. Carers can contribute to safety within the home by reporting anything which is likely to cause an accident and by taking action, wherever possible, to prevent accidents occurring. This will be discussed later in the chapter.

Missing patient

The home should have a policy on action to be taken if a patient goes missing. If the person tends to go out unaccompanied, staff should ask that the individual carries identification in case of accident. A note tucked into a wallet or purse saying 'Mrs Doris Swan is a resident of Eastways Residential Home, in case of accident please telephone....' will help ensure that the home is contacted if an accident occurs.

If the older person tends to wander and may have left the home in a confused state, the home should have a policy for dealing with this. Normally such a policy involves both calling the police and staff searching for the older person. It is possible for the individual to get some distance from the home very quickly. An older person dressed in ordinary clothes will not attract any attention. Many bus drivers do not ask to see bus passes when a person is obviously above retirement age. The police will find it difficult to locate a lady of 83 with white hair and glasses wearing a flowered Marks and Spencer's dress!

Many homes now take photographs of patients. A photograph is often attached to the medication chart to enable staff to identify patients. In some homes photographs of patients are put on their bedroom doors. This helps patients, visitors and staff to find a person's room. If the person goes missing and the police have a recent photograph, their job becomes much easier.

Accidents

Preventing accidents

Carers can contribute to safety within the home by reporting anything which is likely to cause an accident, and by taking action wherever possible to prevent accidents occurring. Some factors which can cause or contribute to accidents are given here.

Environmental hazards

A wet floor can be slippery and can cause a fall. A toilet which is dark because the light bulb does not work and has not been replaced can make it difficult for the person to see where he is going and can cause a fall. A building which is poorly maintained can lead to accidents. Equipment which is not working properly can also cause accidents.

If the carer discovers that the brakes on a patient's wheelchair are not working she should remove the wheelchair and report the problem so that repairs can be organized quickly. Homes should have a spare wheelchair which can be used by staff to transport patients who are ill, or can be used temporarily by a patient whose wheelchair is unsafe.

Objects left carelessly on the floor may not be noticed by older people who can fall over. Carers who notice any hazards which could lead to accidents should remove the hazards wherever possible and inform the person in charge of the home at once.

Inadequate seating can lead to some disabled people falling out of chairs. Some older people living in nursing homes are very disabled and are unable to sit in ordinary armchairs. It is now possible to buy chairs specially designed to enable these people to sit comfortably in chairs that will support them. An example of one of these is given in Fig. 6.1a. Specially designed chairs pro-

Fig. 6.1(a) A Kirton chair, an example of a chair specially designed for frail patients. The cushion slopes backwards to prevent the person falling out of the chair.

Fig. 6.1(b)   Patient seated in a special chair.

vide support for disabled older people but do not restrain or restrict the person in any way (Fig. 6.1b).

Unsuitable footwear

Unsuitable footwear can make it difficult for older people to walk and can lead to accidents. Many older people, especially those who have not been walking around, find that their feet swell. This can make it difficult to find shoes which fit properly. Some older people have deformed feet; bunions and arthritis can cause foot deformities. These deformities can make it very difficult for older people to find shoes which fit properly. Special shoes can be made for patients who have difficulty in wearing ordinary shoes. The patient's GP writes to the surgical fitter (known as an orthotist) and asks for shoes to be made for the patient. The orthotist visits, measures the person's feet, and discusses which type and colour of shoes or boots the person would prefer. These are made specially and the orthotist returns to fit them when they are ready.

Some older people, particularly those who have suffered from strokes, require a calliper to provide support. These are supplied by the orthotist. Sometimes special shoes are made and the calliper is designed to fit into the heel of the shoe. In other cases the older person's own shoes are adapted so that the calliper will fit.

People who suffer from arthritis of the knee may find that one of their knees tends to 'give'. If this is the case a knee support may be required. The orthotist can supply this. People who have broken a leg may have one leg shorter than the other as a result of surgery. Special shoes can be made to correct this and enable the older person to walk normally.

If the older person has been supplied with special footwear or an aid such as a calliper, the carer should help the person to put this on if help is required. Older people who have suitable footwear are less likely to have accidents.

Clothing

Clothing can cause accidents. Many older women prefer full length nightdresses and dressing gowns. If these are too long the individual can trip over and fall. Many male patients wear pyjamas and can easily fall if the legs are too long.

How accidents affect older people

Accidents can have serious consequences. The older person can lose confidence because of a fall and this can cause the individual to walk less and to become weaker. Sometimes the older person who falls fractures a bone. If the person puts out a hand to save himself the wrist may fracture. This is known as a *Colles' fracture*. The thigh bones (femurs) or the top of the thigh bone (shaft of femur) can become fractured as a result of a fall.

Older people often suffer from a condition known as *osteoporosis*. Osteoporosis causes the bones to become thinner and weaker and more easily broken. Figs. 6.2 and 6.3 show healthy bone and bone where osteoporosis has weakened the bone.

Discovering which patients are at risk of having accidents

People living within homes have a wide range of abilities. Some have few problems in walking whilst others require aids and the help of carers to move around. Some patients are alert whilst others are not. Some patients see well whilst others have very poor vision. Some of the people living in your home will be much more likely to have accidents than others.

Homes aim to enable older people to live their lives as they

Fig. 6.2 Normal healthy
bone (enlarged).

Fig. 6.3 Osteoporotic
bone (enlarged).

would wish if they were at home. The aim of care within homes
should be to reduce the risk of accidents and to protect individuals
who are at risk of having accidents. Many homes now have a
policy of assessing if individuals are at risk of having accidents. If
the person is at risk then this is noted in the care plan along with
action to be taken to reduce risks. It is important that carers realise
that no home can be made totally safe and that no one can
guarantee that accidents will not happen.

Balancing risks and quality of life

Living is about taking risks. We all take risks every day of our lives.
We risk crossing the road where there are no traffic lights; we take
risks every time we step into a car or on a bus, or take part in
sports. Yet if we stayed at home and took no risks life would not be
worth living. When we take risks we weigh up the risk and decide
on the possible gains and losses from taking that risk.

In homes staff must balance the duty of care and the possibility
of trying so hard to avoid accidents that we risk making the older
person's life a misery by preventing her from living life to the full.
The carer who left a confused patient alone and unsupervised in
the bath knowing that she was not capable of calling for help
would be failing in her duty of care. Another individual recovering
from illness might ask the carer to sit with her while she bathes
because she is feeling nervous. Another individual might wish to
bath in private and may ask the carer to leave after he has been
helped into the bath.

It is important that the carer does not treat all the patients in the home in the same way. The carer must recognize that older people are just like us, only older, and that they wish to be treated as individuals. Some older people who are recovering from illness are determined to 'get back on their feet'. In the process of regaining mobility and strength the person may fall many times. Staff should respect the individual's wishes and offer support, help and encouragement.

Restraint

It is illegal to restrain any one without their consent. It is also illegal to restrain any person on another person's instructions. In homes carers may see different types of restraint used, including cotsides, tables and lockers.

Cotsides

Cotsides were used routinely in hospitals until a few years ago. Some hospitals had policies which stated that all individuals over a certain age were to have cotsides fitted to their beds to prevent falls. It is now known that cotsides can lead to serious injury and they are only used in special circumstances.

Cotsides prevent individuals getting up, and this can lead to incontinence. When cotsides are used some older people become depressed and upset, and this can affect their mental and physical health and lead to them becoming weaker and sicker. Some people climb over cotsides and can fall. There have been reports of people who caught an arm or leg in the cotside, struggled to get free and broke a limb. The cotside, which is designed to prevent accidents, can actually cause them.

Tables, chairs and lockers

These can be used to barricade the person into bed making it difficult or impossible to get out, but using furniture in this way can lead to accidents.

Preventing the older person falling out of bed

Staff often worry that if a person falls the staff will be blamed and everyone will think the patient has been neglected. Homes which have risk assessment policies will have these documented and patients, staff, relatives and registration officers will be aware of these policies. Older people do not normally fall out of bed and many staff worry unnecessarily about them doing so. Carers can reduce the risk of accidents at night by:

- making sure that the patient can reach the call bell
- assuring the person that staff are there to help and not to hesitate to ring if help is required
- answering bells promptly
- making sure the person does not feel rushed or a 'nuisance'
- leaving a light on so that if the person wishes to get up in the night, he can see
- leaving the room tidy and not leaving any obstacles which could cause a fall
- leaving any aids such as a walking frame and shoes where the person can reach them

In the home where I work the number of accidents has fallen since these measures were introduced and cotsides used only as a last resort.

Recording accidents

All accidents which occur in the home must be recorded in an accident book. The type of record kept varies from area to area. There are no national guidelines stating that homes should maintain these records. In practice accident records which satisfy the local inspection team are kept. In some areas a form is issued in triplicate; one form is kept in the patient's notes, another in an accident folder and another is placed in the care plan. In other areas all accidents are recorded in a bound book. Find out the policy for recording accidents in your home.

Learning from accidents

Some accidents which occur could, with hindsight, have been prevented. In other cases, perhaps involving faulty equipment or poor lifting techniques, accidents may recur if action is not taken. In some homes senior staff discuss and review accidents so that, wherever possible, lessons can be learnt and further accidents prevented.

Medical emergencies

All staff working in care homes come face to face with emergency situations from time to time. Although trained staff are on duty at all times in nursing homes, it is important that you have some basic knowledge of first aid. The aims of first aid are to:

- preserve life
- prevent the emergency worsening
- help recovery

What to do if you find a patient has collapsed

- first take a deep breath and remain calm
- use the call bell to call for help
- check what is happening – is the patient conscious or unconscious? How serious is the situation:

The most important things you can do can be remembered by 'ABC'. Ensure that the person's:

- **A**irway is open and he is able to breath
- **B**reathing is taking place
- **C**irculation is satisfactory

Airway obstruction

The airway enables us to breathe air in and out of our lungs. It can become obstructed for a number of reasons, but the commonest causes of airway obstruction are choking or loss of consciousness.

If the person is choking this could be because food or dentures are blocking the airway. The person may have vomited and vomit has collected at the back of the throat. Open the person's mouth gently. Use two fingers to feel around for any food, vomit or dentures which may be causing the person to choke. Remove anything which is blocking the airway.

If the person is unable to speak and is turning blue use the Heimlich manoeuvre which is shown in Fig. 6.4.

There are many reasons for loss of consciousness, including strokes, fits and diabetes. Carers who know as much about the older person's condition as possible can respond more effectively. People who become unconscious should be placed in the recovery position (Fig. 6.5). You may require help to place a person in this position. If possible remove the person's dentures as they may slip in the mouth and block the airway. Loosen tight clothing and call for help immediately.

Breathing

Some older people suffer from asthma and carry inhalers which help them to breathe more easily. It is important that you find out whether any of the people in the home where you work suffer from asthma. If a person in the home does suffer from asthma and may require help to use an inhaler if he or she has become breathless, find out how to do this before an emergency occurs.

If the person is having difficulty breathing but is conscious, help him to sit up. Loosen any tight clothing, such as a tie, shirt collar or belt. People who have difficulty breathing feel very frightened and this fear makes breathing more difficult. Do your best to reassure

Fig. 6.4 Heimlich manoeuvre.

the person as this will help prevent breathing problems worsening. Ask the person to take slow deep breaths, and seek assistance.

Circulation
If a person becomes unconscious it is important for the carer to be able to decide quickly if the situation is a life threatening emergency or simply a faint:

- check the person's colour – blue or grey skin indicates a life threatening emergency
- check breathing – is the person breathing at all, with difficulty or normally
- check the pulse – is the pulse absent or does it appear weak

Tilt head back

Place hand beneath head for support

Bend arm for stable positioning

Bend leg to support the body and stop the patient rolling forward

Fig. 6.5   Recovery position.

If the person's skin colour is abnormal or breathing is absent, or the person is breathing with difficulty, or the pulse is absent or weak, call for help immediately. This is a medical emergency perhaps caused by a stroke or heart attack. Check that the airway is clear and place the person in the recovery position whilst waiting for help.

Fainting is a brief loss of consciousness. People who have fainted may appear very pale but their skin does not become blue or grey. Breathing is normal and the pulse is always present, though it can appear weak. Fainting can occur in adults of all ages. It may be caused by hunger, shock, or even getting up too quickly. The person faints because the brain is not receiving sufficient blood. A person who has fainted should not be sat up because sitting up reduces the flow of blood to the brain.

If you find a person unconscious, it is important to check their colour. Clothing should be loosened and the person should lie down until she feels well enough to sit up. Drinking from a glass of cold water may help the person to feel better.

Chest pain

Chest pain and circulation problems can be caused by *angina* or a *heart attack*. In both cases the heart muscle will not be getting sufficient blood and oxygen. If the person is unconscious, place them in the recovery position. If they are conscious help them to breathe by sitting them up and loosening clothing. *Call for help at once.*

If the person is known to have a heart condition his GP may have prescribed tablets or a spray of the drug glycerine trinitrate. This drug acts by helping the arteries that bring blood to the heart to expand, which improves the supply of blood to the heart.

Check if any of the patients in the home where you work are known to have a heart condition. If anyone has been prescribed glycerine trinitrate by a GP find out how this is given in an emergency *before* the emergency occurs.

Bleeding

Bleeding can be caused by a fall. If the patient is bleeding remain calm. A clean towel or item of clothing can be applied to the wound and pressure applied to control bleeding. A sterile dressing pack can be fetched when help arrives, and the wound can be cleaned and examined to decide what further treatment is required.

Suspected fractures

The aim of first aid is to prevent movement of the injured part of the body and to arrange for the person to be transferred to hospital as soon as possible. In some cases it is obvious that a person has fractured and patients with obvious fractures are sent to hospital at once by ambulance. Before dialling 999 for an ambulance ask:

- What happened?
- Where is the pain:

The ambulance staff answering the emergency call will require this information.

If you have any suspicion that the person has fractured do not move them. Ambulance para-medics will support the limb before moving the person

- do not give the person anything to eat or drink, as emergency surgery may be required
- it is important to keep the person warm – place a blanket over them
- if the person is bleeding, apply direct pressure to the wound to control bleeding

Burns and scalds

Burns are caused by dry heat; scalds are caused by hot liquids. The treatment of burns and scalds is the same. The aims of first aid in this case are to:

- stop the pain
- relieve pain and swelling
- prevent infection

Carers should:

- assess the severity of the burn and call for professional help
- place the burnt area under cold running water for at least ten minutes
- if the hand has been burnt remove rings and watches if possible
- do not try to remove clothing which may be stuck to the skin
- do not apply any creams to the burn
- do not burst blisters
- do not apply a dressing to the burn – these may stick and cause further damage
- if the burn is severe the skin can be wrapped in cling film or placed in a clean plastic bag until help arrives

Learning more about first aid

All carers should have some basic knowledge of first aid. If you are working in a residential home in a senior capacity, you will require training to equip you with the skills needed to cope in an emergency. Carers working in nursing homes may also benefit from such training. The St John Ambulance run first aid courses locally and further details can be obtained from:

Medical Department
St John Ambulance
1 Grosvenor Crescent
London SW1X 7EF.
Telephone 0171 235 5231

Summary

Staff working in homes should aim to provide an environment which is as safe as possible for older people. There is, however, no such thing as a 'safe' environment. Staff should work with older people and support them in living their lives as they wish. Many homes have policies which help determine the risk of people falling or having accidents. Accidents should be recorded and where possible action should be taken to prevent similar accidents occurring.

Caring for the older person's possessions

People living in homes may ask staff to look after possessions for them. The home should have a policy on looking after money and valuables for patients. Some older people ask their families to look after possessions whilst others prefer to leave these at home. Some older people living in homes do not have any family and friends and rely on staff to help them look after possessions.

Older people living in homes whose fees are paid by either social services under the Community Care Act (1990) or who have their fees met by the Department of Social Security (DSS) under earlier funding arrangements, are entitled to a 'personal allowance'. This allowance is £13.15 per week in 1995, and is to enable older people to buy clothing and other items which they may require.

Keeping records of patients' money

Homes are obliged to keep a record of any money which they look after for older people. In many homes patients ask staff to buy things for them at the shops. Whenever possible older people should be encouraged to accompany staff to the shops and given the opportunity to select and buy things themselves. When staff buy things for patients a full record of the money spent should be kept. This protects patients from financial abuse and protects staff from any accusations of theft. An example of such a record is given in Fig. 6.6.

Name: *Mrs Daisy Brown*   Room: *4*

Date	Income Description	Amount	Outgoings Description	Balance
20/4/95	*Pension*	*£13.15*		
22/4/95			*Toiletries £3*	*£10.15*
23/4/95			*Chocolates £2.50*	*£7.65*
27/4/95	*Pension*	*£13.15*		*£20.80*
28/4/95			*Perm £15*	*£5.80*

Fig. 6.6   Patient's personal money log.

Keeping records of other items left for safekeeping

Staff may be asked to keep other items for the patient. A record of this should be kept. This may be a note in the patient's progress notes or it may be written in a book kept for this purpose, normally known as a patient's property or valuables book. Carers should be careful about recording items. All that glitters is not gold and all white stones that sparkle are not diamonds; the carer should record 'one yellow metal ring with a white stone' not 'gold ring with diamond solitaire'.

Patients who retain valuable items

Some older people wear valuable items and do not wish to leave them in the home's safe. They have every right to continue to wear valuable items of jewellery. Imagine how you would feel if your treasured engagement ring or locket was taken away and locked in a safe in case you lose it. If the older person is wearing rings or has brought jewellery into the home a note of this should be made. Many homes state that they cannot take responsibility for items which have been lost unless a robbery has taken place. In some homes patients can take out an insurance policy to insure against losing valuables.

It is important that relatives and staff communicate well. Staff in countless homes have spent hours searching for 'lost' rings only to discover later that relatives have taken them to jewellers to have them adjusted because they no longer fit. In the home where I work, several staff spent hours searching for a ring which a forgetful patient had misplaced. We found the ring finally in the dustbag in the vacuum cleaner. Later we discovered that the ring we thought we were searching for, which had been in the older person's family for over a hundred years, had in fact been replaced with a copy by the patient's family with her consent. The patient had forgotten to tell us and so had the relatives.

Precious items

Some items such as spectacles, hearing aids and dentures have no value to anyone except their owner. Carers should ensure that they help older people to keep track of such possessions. If such items are lost and cannot be found, replacement should be organized. Spectacles can be engraved with the owner's surname or initials by many opticians. Dentures and hearing aids can also be engraved with the person's name if required. This engraving can be done discreetly and enables carers to identify possessions which have been left behind perhaps in the lounge or dining room.

Portfolio preparation

- Ask if you can take a copy of the home's health and safety policy for your portfolio.
- Prepare details on fire training you have received.

- Ask if you can take a copy of any policies which the home has on missing patients.
- Include details of how money and valuables are safeguarded in the home.
- Find out if the home's insurance policy insures patients' personal effects.
- If your home has a risk assessment policy to decide which patients are at risk of accidents, include this in your portfolio.
- If the home has a restraint policy include this.
- Give details of any instruction you have received to enable you to cope with emergencies.

Further information

Health & Safety at Work Act (1974) HMSO, London. Your home will probably have a copy of the Act; if not the local reference library or your college library will have one.

Fire safety. The local fire station will have a number of videos which you may find of interest. Fire brigade staff use these when giving talks to various groups. One video which you may find interesting is *Hospitals don't just burn down.* This video was made about 16 years ago but is still useful. The fire station may lend you this video but will require identification before doing so.

Fire Safety Services
Low Burnham Hall
Halgarth
Nr Epworth
Doncaster DN9 1DE.
Telephone 01427 874294

Fire Safety Services have released a training video aimed at staff working in nursing and residential homes. Your home or college may have one which you can borrow.

Further reading

St John Ambulance, British Red Cross Society and St Andrew's Ambulance Association (1994) *First Aid Manual*, 6th edn. Dorling Kindersley, London.
Counsel & Care (1993) *The Right to Take Risks*. Counsel & Care, London.

Chapter 7

Record Keeping and Confidentiality

Introduction

This chapter gives details on how information is collected and stored within the home and how confidentiality is maintained. This includes:

- pre-admission assessments
- legal requirements – which records must be kept
- care plans and progress notes
- who writes care plans and progress notes
- medical records storage and access
- maintaining confidentiality
- dealing with relatives
- telephone enquiries

The importance of communication

Most staff working in homes work shifts. It is important that information relating to the care of older people living in the home is recorded. Recording information enables all staff to ensure that the care given is of the highest quality. Carers work closely with older people and the person may confide in or discuss her condition with the carer. If the carer passes on that information to other staff, this can improve the quality of care. Older people depend on the staff working within homes, and staff have a duty to act in a professional way and protect the confidentiality of information which they gain in the course of their work.

Assessments

In recent years most homes have developed a system which entails assessing the patient before admission. An example of a patient assessment sheet is given in Fig. 7.1. Assessments are normally carried out by a senior member of staff. In residential homes this

PATIENT ASSESSMENT SHEET

Name:	Room Permanent/Temporary
Address:	D.O.B. Age Date/Time admitted:
	Accompanied by:
Tel No:	
Marital Status:	Type of Admission: Emergency Waiting List
Religion:	
Next of Kin:	Reason for Admission:
Relationship:	
Address:	Confirmed Diagnosis:
Tel No:	
Contact in Emergency:	Patient aware of reason for admission:
G.P.	Urinalysis Weight:
Address:	
Tel No:	Past Medial History *(serious illnesses & hospitalisation)*
Lives alone: Yes/No	
Property: *if any valuables are stored, state what and where*	
Discharge/Transfer	
When:	
Where to:	Allergies:
Transport:	
Reason:	
TTAS:	Investigations and Date:
Relatives informed	
General Appearance:	Vision:
Mobility–help needed	Elimination:
Walking Dressing	Urinary:
Bathing Eating	
Comments:	Bowel:
Mental State:	Nutritional State:
Comments:	Dietary Preferences:
	Special Diet:
Skin State:	Sleep:
Broken Areas:	Usual Pattern
Norton Score:	Sedation
Oral Inspection:	Pain–Description:
Dentures Full/Partial	
Hearing:	Leisure Activities, Interests:
Uses Aid	
	History taken by:
	From:

Fig. 7.1   Patient assessment sheet.

will be the manager. In nursing homes the matron, deputy matron or a senior RGN will carry out the assessment.

The person assessing will visit the older person, who may be living at home, in a residential home (if nursing home admission is being considered) or may be in hospital. The aims of assessment are to meet the older person and to check that the home can meet the individual's care needs. If the manager of a residential home discovers that the older person has nursing needs, the manager may suggest that a nursing home is more appropriate. Under current legislation residential homes should provide the type of care which would be given by a caring relative at home.

If the older person is extremely confused, with a long history of dementia, and may leave the home and be at risk of being run over on the busy road outside the home, the matron may suggest that the individual requires care in a nursing home registered for the elderly mentally infirm. In such a home the individual would benefit from the care of nurses trained to meet the person's mental health needs.

If the person assessing feels that the home can meet the patient's care needs, the assessment gives both the older person and the member of staff the opportunity to meet and discuss the home. If possible the older person should visit the home, but if they are recovering from an illness in hospital this is not always possible and relatives or friends may visit on the person's behalf.

Next time someone from your home is visiting an older person to carry out an assessment, ask if you can go. This will give you an opportunity to watch an assessment and get to know the older person before admission. The information obtained at assessment enables the assessor to begin to plan care.

Patient records

Homes are required to maintain certain records under the Registered Homes Act 1984[1]. This Act sets out how homes should be run in England, Wales and Northern Ireland. In Scotland the Registered Homes Act 1939 is the relevant Act of Parliament. Under both Acts homes are required to keep admission records, records of accidents and a daily record of patient treatment.

Admission records

Homes are required to keep a register of all patients admitted to the home. This should include details of the patient's name, address, place admitted from (for example a local hospital), GP's name, the address and telephone numbers of the next of kin and the date of admission. The date of discharge or death should be entered when the patient leaves the home.

In residential homes care assistants will normally fill in the admission register. In most nursing homes it has become viewed as the responsibility of trained staff, although the reasons for this are unclear. In hospitals the admission register may be filled in by the ward clerk or a care assistant or a trained nurse.

Ask if your home has a policy on who can complete the admission register. Perhaps the trained staff would welcome help in completing paperwork when a patient is admitted.

These records must be retained by law for one year after the last entry. Many homes retain these records for seven years after the last entry.

Daily statements of patient's health

Homes are required by law to keep a daily statement of patient's health. One record of the patient's health must be entered every 24 hours by law. In practice most homes write in the patient's records twice in 24 hours. One record is normally made by the day staff and one by the night staff. The Registered Homes Acts are both rather old and there are plans to review them and introduce new legislation in 1996. The Acts do not specify the type of records to be kept.

Care plans

In the past, patient care was planned on the basis of 'task allocation'. Each member of the team was allocated tasks which took account of the abilities of that member of staff. One member of staff might have been asked to check all the patient's temperatures, pulses and blood pressures. Another two members of staff might have been asked to make all the beds. This system of care had several drawbacks. The first was that patients were cared for by many different staff and few patients got to know staff. Also, staff felt as if they were working on a production line and that they had little opportunity to get to know patients. Using a task allocation system meant that most patients with the same condition were treated in exactly the same way.

The system now used in most homes is that of individualized patient care. This system aims to treat the person as an individual. Two people who have arthritis in the knees may have entirely different priorities and needs. Mrs Caine, for example, may have difficulty in walking because of her arthritis and this may be preventing her from attending church on Sundays. Mr Edwards may find that the pain in his knees is preventing him from getting a good night's sleep.

The basis of individualized care is the care plan. This plan is drawn up in consultation with the patient. In nursing homes trained nurses use a 'nursing model' to help them draw up the care plan. There are a number of nursing models and one commonly used was drawn up by Roper, Logan and Tierney[2]. This model identifies twelve activities of daily living (Fig. 7.2). The nurse uses these activities to help plan care.

---

1. Maintaining a safe environment
2. Communication
3. Breathing
4. Eating and drinking
5. Eliminating
6. Personal cleansing and dressing
7. Controlling body temperature
8. Mobilizing
9. Sleeping
10. Religious needs
11. Social activity
12. Expressing sexuality
13. Wounds and dressings
14. Dying

The nurse may identify other needs.

Fig. 7.2   Activities of daily living (Roper, Logan & Tierney 1990).

The care plan is used to identify the patient's needs, the aims of nursing care, the action which is taken to help meet these needs and the outcome of the care. A copy of a care plan is shown in Fig. 7.3.

Information recorded on a care plan

The care plan contains information about the person's day to day care.

It should give details of any assistance required to wash or bathe; this may include using a bath hoist. It will also include the person's preferences, for example if the person prefers to bath or shower.

It should give details of the person's mobility. If the person uses a frame to walk this should be recorded. If the person requires a walking aid and the help of one or two members of staff to walk, this will be recorded.

Date	Needs	Aim	Action	Evaluation
23/6/95	To keep	To help	1) Walk with Mrs Morris	
	clean and	Mrs Morris	to bathroom	
①	fresh	bathe and	2) Use hoist to help her	
		wash	get into bath	
			3) Help Mrs Morris wash	
			her back and feet	
			4) Leave Mrs Morris to	
			soak if she wishes	
			5) Ensure Mrs Morris	
			can reach call bell	
②	To walk	1) To help	1) Help to put caliper	
	independently	Mrs Morris	on left leg	
		remain able	2) Assist with putting	
		to walk	on shoes	
		independently	3) Ensure Mrs Morris's	
			tripod is within easy	
			reach	

Name: Mrs Edna Morris   Room No: 2   Age: 92

Fig. 7.3 Sample care plan.

If the person has a continence problem this should be recorded. A separate continence assessment will also have been undertaken and this will be kept separately. Treatment to promote continence such as a toileting programme or bladder retraining will be noted on the care plan.

If the older person requires a special diet, has difficulty in feeding herself or requires aids to enable her to feed herself, this will be noted on the care plan.

The care plan should identify the person's needs and the aims of care, and give details of how that care is to be given. After a time the effectiveness of the care given will be evaluated.

Carers should read the older person's care plan so that they are aware of the care required and the reasons that this particular care is given. A carer might think that it is cruel to expect a person who has recently had surgery to repair a fractured femur to begin walking again. The care plan should explain the reasons why the older person should be encouraged to walk again.

Carers can often help trained staff give better care by informing them of how the person is feeling. The individual may tell the carer that she wishes to walk but is still having a lot of pain. The individual may not have told the trained nurse about this pain, even though the nurse has asked. The individual may not wish to 'bother' the nurse. If the carer informs the nurse, arrangements can be made to ensure that the patient receives satisfactory pain relief. In this way nurses and carers can work together to ensure that the older person receives care of the highest quality.

Sometimes trained nurses use technical terms which the carer may not understand. Throughout this book I have given technical terms and explained them to enable carers to understand care plans more fully. Nursing staff sometimes use abbreviations and initials and these can appear confusing to carers. If you do not understand terms or abbreviations used in nursing records ask the nursing staff. They will usually be only too pleased to explain and will be delighted that you are keen to learn.

Progress report

A progress report (Fig. 7.4) is used as a daily record of the individual's care. The information recorded in the progress notes goes from home to home. Check the policy in your home about what is recorded in the patient's progress notes.

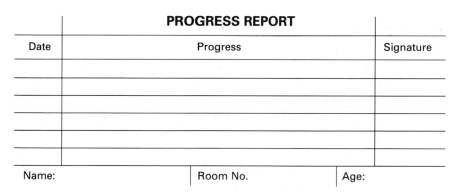

Fig. 7.4   Sample of a progress report sheet.

Who writes care plans and progress notes

Some residential homes now employ qualified staff. Although under the terms of the Nursing Homes Acts trained nurses are not to use their nursing skills in residential homes, in practice many do. If the residential home you are working in employs a qualified nurse or a number of qualified nurses they may write the care plans and progress notes. In residential homes where qualified nursing staff are not employed the care assistants will be responsible for writing care plans and maintaining progress notes. These will be less detailed than those kept by nursing homes because the people living in residential homes will require less care.

If a person living in a residential home is being visited by a district nurse, perhaps to treat a leg ulcer, the district nurse may write in the care plan. If the person is receiving therapy from another professional, such as speech therapy, the speech therapist may wish to write in the care plan. The speech therapist may write instructions and advice which help carers continue to help the person make progress with speech between treatments. The policy will vary from home to home. Find out what the policy is in your home.

In nursing homes the policy will also vary from home to home. In large homes which have several qualified nurses on each shift, all records may be kept by qualified nurses. The qualified nurse will normally discuss the care of any patient with the carer who has given the care. The qualified nurse will then complete the report. If the carer is aware of any changes in the person's condition or if the older person has told the carer something of which the qualified nurse is not aware, the carer should inform the trained nurse.

The carer may be helping the individual to get up after an afternoon nap and notices that the person appears pale and faint. The carer can then inform the qualified nurse who may suspect that the new tablets the patient's doctor has prescribed for her blood pressure are causing problems. The qualified nurse is then aware of the problem and can investigate and take further action.

In some homes carers may be asked to fill in the progress reports. Any entry is checked by the qualified nurse who countersigns the entry. In this situation carers should be instructed and helped to fill in such reports by the qualified nurse. Check the procedure in your home. In nursing homes other professionals such as physiotherapists, speech therapists, nurses specializing in the care of people with diabetes or continence advisers, will be frequent visitors. This is because older people who live in nursing homes require greater levels of skilled care than those living in residential homes. In many homes these professionals will write in the care plan.

Further records stored in the home

People living in homes have other records. When the older person is admitted to the home a letter is normally sent from the person's GP, if the person was admitted from home. If the person was admitted from hospital, a note will have been sent to the home. If the person's GP has asked other professionals, such as a physiotherapist, speech therapist or clinical nurse specialist, to treat the patient, he will write a referral letter.

Details of inpatient visits whilst living in the home will also need to be stored. Old care plans, medication charts and other papers will require storage. In many homes a folder is made up and all these records are stored in the folder. Many GPs also write notes about the treatment they prescribe and keep them in this folder. Although GPs keep separate records detailing patient treatment, many also keep notes at the home. GPs prefer to do this in case the patient needs to be seen by another doctor in an emergency or patient records are required by hospital staff. These records are normally stored in a locked cupboard or filing cabinet in the home, to protect confidentiality.

Access to medical and nursing records

Patients now have a legal right to have access to their health records under the Access to Medical Records Act [3] which became law in 1990. The patient writes to the doctor who is providing care, normally the older person's GP in homes, and requests copies of all records.

Nursing homes are inspected by registration and inspection officers employed by the local NHS Trust. Residential homes are inspected by inspection officers employed by social services. Inspection officers have the power to ask to see day to day records relating to care. They do not have the right to see medical records unless the inspector is a qualified medical practitioner.

Patient confidentiality

Staff who work with older people learn a great deal about those they care for. All staff must ensure that information which they discover in the course of their work remains confidential. Most carers are very aware of how essential it is to maintain confidentiality at all times; however, staff can inadvertently betray confidentiality. This may occur in the following situations:

- discussing the patient's condition with another member of staff within earshot of other patients or relatives
- in conversation outside of work, perhaps at the bus stop, on a train or in a restaurant or pub, where this conversation may be overheard by others
- by using the patient's name in NVQ evidence gathering – normally initials are used to maintain confidentiality

■ by leaving patient records lying around – the nursing notes or other records may be left where other patients have access to them

■ by disclosing information about the person's condition to relatives and friends without their consent.

It is important that carers are always aware of the need to maintain confidentiality, as the relationship between carer and patient is built on trust. Betraying that trust may destroy the caring relationship.

Dealing with relatives

Many relatives will approach carers, even junior members of staff who have not been working in the home for very long, and ask how the patient is. It is important that the carer finds out the home's policy on giving information to relatives. Carers who have worked in hospital before may have been told to refer all queries to qualified nurses. In homes the policy will be different. In most homes the enquiry is partly a way of starting a conversation with the carer and only a general answer is required. For example Mrs Jenkin's daughter might say:

'Hello Julie, I've come to see Mum. How is she today?'

In this case the carer would reply, 'Well, she's just had her hair done and she's been looking forward to your visit.'

In other cases the relative might be asking for more specific information, but the carer can deal with this; for example, Mrs Franklin's daughter asks:

'How did mum get on at the opticians when she had her eyes tested?'

The carer might reply, 'The optician said she needs new glasses so she's chosen the frames and they should be ready on Tuesday.'

In other cases the carer may not have the information or may not be able to answer the relative's questions fully and should ask the qualified nurse or the home's manager to speak to the relative; for example, Mrs Davis's daughter asks:

'How did mum get on down at the hospital when she saw the specialist about her arthritic hip?'

The carer might reply, 'I think the specialist spoke to Sister James about her hip. If you hold on I'll just see if I can find her and she can have a word with you.'

In each of these examples the carer has given the relative as much information and help as possible. The carer has shown the relative that she is aware of the patient's treatment but is not getting out of her depth and attempting to give information which she does not completely understand.

Telephone queries

In many homes the matron or manager answers the telephone whenever possible and deals with telephone queries. When the person in charge is busy other staff often answer the telephone. It is important to state the name of the home and your name when answering, for example 'High Trees Nursing Home, Penny Jones speaking,' or 'care assistant Jones speaking'. This helps maintain the home's professional image. Always find out who is calling, and if the person is asking to speak to the person in charge ask the nature of their call. If the sister in charge of the nursing home is attending to a patient who is ill and she is aware that the call is from the representative of a company selling cleaning products, she can give you a message to tell them to call back at a more convenient time.

Many relatives and friends telephone to ask how patients are. This is often just a general enquiry, for example:
'This is Mrs Gibson. How is my mum, Mrs Kelly, today?'
'She's fine; all her birthday cards have arrived and she's opening them now.'
'Can you tell her we'll pick her up at 1 o'clock and take her out to lunch?'
If Mrs Kelly was unwell, the carer would fetch the person in charge who could speak to the relative.

Many homes have a policy about who should answer the telephone, who should give certain information and under what circumstances this information is given. Many homes do not tell relatives over the telephone that a person has died, unless the older person has been ill and the death is expected. Find out policies in your home on relaying information over the telephone. If the carer is unsure of what to say in certain circumstances she should ask a more senior member of staff to take the call.

Portfolio preparation

- Find out if your home has a written policy on confidentiality. Ask if you can copy it and include it in your portfolio.
- Find out who has access to records and include details in your portfolio.
- Include details of your role within the home in giving information to senior staff and to relatives.
- Outline how you maintain confidentiality while carrying out your work.

Summary

Homes store a variety of records relating to the medical and nursing care of the older people living in the home. Some of this information is extremely sensitive and disclosure could cause great embarrassment to the older person and could breach the caring relationship between staff and patient. Records should be stored in a safe place and only staff should have access to these records. The older person has the legal right to see these records on request. Older people grow to respect and trust their carers. Carers have a duty to ensure that patient confidentiality is maintained at all times.

References

(1)   Registered Homes Act 1984 (revised 1988). HMSO, London. The home where you work will have a copy of this Act which you can study. Section one relates to residential homes and section two to nursing homes. The Act also has some guidance notes which explain the legal language used in the Act. This is supplied as an appendix to the Act and your home should have a copy of this.

(2)   Roper, Logan & Tierney (1990) *The Elements of Nursing*, 3rd edn. Churchill-Livingstone, Edinburgh.

(3)   Access to Health Records Act (1990). HMSO, London. Your local college may have a copy of this Act in the library. If not you can visit the reference library at your local library, read the Act and take photocopies if you wish.

Chapter 8

Mobility

Introduction

This chapter will provide information on:

- the benefits of remaining mobile
- how illness affects mobility
- the dangers of immobility
- helping older people to remain mobile
- walking aids
- helping and encouraging older people to use aids
- obtaining aids
- helping people to maintain independence in wheelchairs
- transferring from a wheelchair
- exercise and passive movement.

Benefits of remaining mobile

The ability to move around freely is one which we often take for granted. Many older people who enter nursing homes have problems moving around. Some are unable to move unaided from bed to chair and some are bedbound. Some develop deformities which mean that they can no longer straighten arms or legs, and hands may become permanently closed in fists. Professional staff in some homes may explain to carers that such changes are the inevitable effects of ageing and that older people become immobile as a result of ageing.

Whilst older people may become immobile in the last few months or weeks of life, many older people living in nursing and residential homes become immobile because of poorly managed care. It is difficult to find out how long the average older person lives in a nursing or residential home. It is estimated that the average person living in a residential home lives there for four years. Older people are estimated to live in nursing homes for an average of 22 months.

The way staff work within homes may not only prevent some older people from regaining mobility after illness, it can also cause older people to become less mobile and more dependent. The goal of care in nursing and residential homes should be to enable older people to retain and regain mobility. This in turn enables them to retain the ability to care for themselves, and enjoy a superior quality of life within the home. It also reduces staff workload.

This chapter will outline how illness affects the older person's ability to move around, the dangers of immobility, and how carers can help older people to retain independence after illness. Some older people, normally those who are extremely ill or disabled, will require greater levels of assistance and may need to be moved. This is dealt with in Chapter 9.

How illness affects an older person's ability to move around

Many older people are admitted to nursing and residential homes from hospital, although some are admitted from home. Most are admitted because the effects of an accident or illness mean that the individual can no longer manage to care for him or herself at home. Some older people are admitted because a long standing illness has worsened and it is impossible to provide the levels of support and care required at home. Others are admitted because of a sudden illness or an accident.

It is possible for many older people who are unable to care for themselves at home to enjoy life in a home where the support they require is given. There is a danger that staff who are not aware of the older person's abilities may discourage the older person from moving around the home. In other cases older people may require encouragement, help, support and aids to help them walk. It is important that carers are aware of how illness affects an individual's ability to walk, so that they can offer appropriate support and help.

Arthritis

Arthritis is a disease that affects all people as they age. Adults start to develop arthritic changes from the age of 40 onwards. Although all older people have arthritis, not all suffer the symptoms. An estimated 12% of men and 25% of women over the age of 70 suffer pain, stiffness and difficulties in moving because of arthritis. There are two types of arthritis: *osteo-arthritis* and *rheumatoid arthritis*.

Osteo-arthritis

Osteo means bone, and arthritis means damage or inflammation. Osteo-arthritis is damage and inflammation to the bone. The ends of bone at joints are covered with a thin layer of smooth material called cartilage. The end of the bone and the cartilage are surrounded by a thick fluid which is called synovial fluid. This is contained in a thin membrane which is known as the synovial membrane. Cartilage and synovial fluid cushion the end of the bone from the effects of movement and act as shock absorbers. The cartilage becomes thinned and roughened when osteo-arthritis is present. The bone is not so well protected from the shock of movement and thickens, the amount of fluid increases and the joint appears swollen. In severe osteo-arthritis the cartilage can wear away completely and bone can rub on bone. The joints affected usually become visibly deformed. Fig. 8.1 shows a healthy knee joint and Fig. 8.2 shows a knee joint affected by osteo-arthritis.

The causes of osteo-arthritis are not yet known. People are more likely to develop osteo-arthritis as they become older and people who have injured a joint or had an operation on a joint are more likely to develop osteo-arthritis. It often develops in people who have taken part in active sports.

The joints affected are usually the hand, hips, knees and big

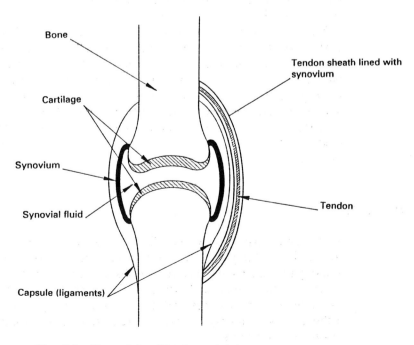

Fig. 8.1 Normal, healthy knee joint.

Inflamed synovium

Thick, abnormal bone with
no remaining cartilage

Distorted, damaged capsule

Loss of remaining cartilage

Fig. 8.2   An osteo-arthritic knee joint.

toes. Osteo-arthritis of the hip usually affects one hip more severely than the other. It can lead to one leg becoming slightly shorter. This can cause walking difficulties and back pain. Osteo-arthritis of the hip is more common in men than in women. Osteo-arthritis of the knee is more common in women.

Osteo-arthritis normally affects only one or two joints. Although many people who suffer from osteo-arthritis find that pain and stiffness is worse in damp weather, dampness does not cause the problem. People all over the world suffer from this condition.

Osteo-arthritis causes pain, stiffness and swelling. The stiffness is made worse by remaining in one position for a long time, and will improve after a few minutes exercise. Pain is normally treated by pain killing tablets, known as analgesics. Aspirin and para-cetamol are commonly prescribed by doctors. If these are not effective, anti-inflammatory drugs are often prescribed. These drugs act not only by treating pain but also by reducing the inflammation in the joint. Such drugs are known as non-steroidal anti-inflammatory drugs.

Overweight people who suffer from osteo-arthritis will feel

much better if they lose weight, because extra weight increases the strain on joints.

Rheumatoid arthritis

Rheumatoid arthritis is an inflammatory disease of the joints. The synovial tissue which covers the joints becomes inflamed. This causes the affected joints to become hot, swollen and painful. Fig. 8.3 shows how rheumatoid arthritis affects a joint. Rheumatoid arthritis normally affects many joints. A person with rheumatoid arthritis may suffer from pain and inflammation in the shoulders, arms, wrists, fingers and toes. Although this is a chronic disease there are often periods when it settles down and causes few problems. At other times the individual suffers an acute attack and joints become very painful. During an acute attack people are advised to rest the joints as much as possible.

In mild cases paracetamol or aspirin are prescribed. In more severe cases non-steroidal anti-inflammatory drugs are prescribed. Doctors may prescribe steroids in severe cases. The cause of rheumatoid arthritis is not yet known.

It is important that people suffering from all types of arthritis keep as active as possible. Many years ago it was thought that the

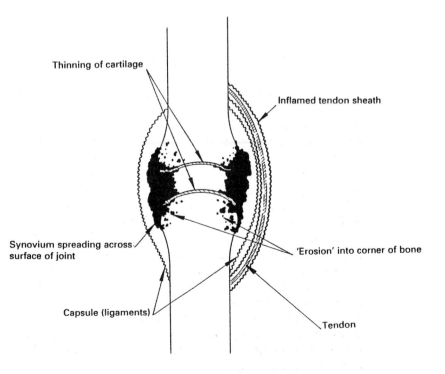

Fig. 8.3 How rheumatoid arthritis affects a joint.

best treatment for all types was rest. Many people with arthritis of all types were admitted to hospital and kept on strict bedrest. Arthritic joints were often put in plaster of Paris casts to prevent any movement. It was thought then that joints became worn out by too much movement. Now people who are suffering from acute rheumatoid arthritis are advised to rest their swollen joints but to take gentle exercise. People suffering from chronic rheumatoid arthritis and osteo-arthritis are advised to carry on with gentle exercise and remain as mobile as possible (Fig 8.4). Some older people worry that exercise will cause further damage to joints, and they need reassurance that this will not happen. Gentle exercise will reduce stiffness and help them to remain as fit as possible.

Fig. 8.4 Patient with arthritic hands using specially adapted cutlery to eat.

Further information

The Arthritis and Rheumatism Council for Research (ARC)
Copeman House
St Mary's Court
Chesterfield
Derbyshire S41 7TD.
Telephone 01246 558033

ARC is a charity which provides information for patients, carers, doctors and nurses. It produces a wide range of leaflets and booklets, including *Rheumatoid Arthritis* – a hand book for patients, and *Osteo-Arthritis* – a booklet for patients. Single copies are available free of charge. ARC will provide full details of their publications on request.

Strokes

Many older people are admitted to homes after suffering from strokes. The medical term for a stroke is a *cerebro-vascular accident*. Nursing and medical staff often refer to this as a CVA.

Normally blood flows around the brain, feeding it with oxygen and sugar (Fig. 8.5). A stroke causes the blood supply to the brain to be interrupted and part of the brain is starved of oxygen. There are two main causes of strokes. Some occur because the blood

Fig. 8.5 Blood flows from the heart to the brain via the arterial circulation.

to break or fracture. This is because of a disease called osteoporosis which is especially common in women.

When older people fall they often break wrists, thigh bones
(femurs) or hips. Nowadays most people who suffer from fractured
femurs have surgical treatment. The bone is pulled together and
held in place with a metal plate and screws. If the neck of the
femur is fractured a screw may be inserted to hold the bone
together, or the surgeon may replace the neck of the femur with
metal. If the hip is fractured the surgeon may carry out a hip
replacement.

Many older people who have fallen over, broken a bone and
undergone major surgery are discharged to homes unable to walk.
This may be because the individual is in a lot of pain following
treatment. Carers should ask such individuals if they are in pain
and inform professional staff so that pain killers may be given.
Some older people who are in pain do not tell staff. One recent
survey carried out in hospital found that patients who were in pain
waited for nursing staff to ask about pain because they did not
want to appear to be complaining. The same survey found that
nursing staff waited for patients to tell them that they were in pain.
The carer should learn to observe individuals, as often our behaviour shows whether we are in pain.

Many older people who have had a severe fall have lost all
confidence in walking. They may require encouragement and help
in beginning to walk again. Some older people who have had
surgery to repair a fractured femur or hip may now have one leg
shorter than the other. This can make walking difficult and dangerous. Fortunately it can easily be corrected by ordering and
providing special shoes. One shoe has a slightly higher, built-up
heel and this corrects any differences in leg length. Further details
are given later in the chapter.

Vision

Poor vision can make it difficult for older people to move around
freely. Research from the Royal College of Opticians shows that
96% of people over the age of 80 require spectacles. Many older
people admitted to nursing and residential homes wear spectacles
but may not have had their eyes tested for many years. New
spectacles and an up to date prescription for lenses may help them
to move around with new found confidence.

Some older people suffer from cataracts. These affect vision
long before they are visible to carers. Now many older people can
benefit from cataract surgery. An eye test will detect the presence
of cataracts.

Some older people suffer from eye diseases such as glaucoma. Untreated glaucoma can cause blindness. An eye test will detect the presence of glaucoma and the patient's doctor can prescribe eye drops which will prevent vision deteriorating.

Some older people suffer from extremely poor vision and little can be done to improve it. If the carer is aware that the individual's vision is poor, she can ensure that the environment is as safe as possible. Details of maintaining a safe environment are given in Chapter 6.

The dangers of immobility

When older people lose the ability to move around freely it has a devastating effect on their physical and mental health. Many older people fear becoming a burden and wish to carry on caring for themselves. The idea of being dependent on others is very upsetting to them. Imagine what it must be like to be unable to walk to the toilet and to have to rely on others to take you. Imagine how it must feel to be unable to get up when you wish or to go to bed when you wish. Many older people become depressed, anxious and upset when they lose the ability to move around.

The physical effects of immobility are also distressing. People who sit for long periods often find that their feet and ankles become swollen. This is because they are not walking. Walking helps the veins to return blood to the heart. People who are sitting for long periods are at risk of developing blood clots in the legs. These are called *deep vein thrombosis*. A deep vein thrombosis can break away from the vein in the leg and enter the venous circulation. The clot then travels around the body until it becomes stuck either in a heart valve or in the vein entering the lung (pulmonary vein). This condition is known as a *pulmonary embolism* and can be fatal.

Moving around causes us to breathe more deeply and this deep breathing is one of the things which protects us against chest infections. People who are immobile are more at risk of developing a chest infection than those who walk around.

Movement causes the bowel to contract. People who do not move around are more at risk of becoming constipated. People who can go to the toilet without help are less likely to suffer from incontinence than those who require help. People who require help are dependent on staff to take them to the toilet. Often staff do not respond quickly enough to an individual's call for assistance (perhaps because they are doing something else) and incontinence can result. People who are not using muscles find that their muscles quickly become smaller and weaker and strength and ability is rapidly lost.

Helping older people to move around

The role of carers in helping individuals to retain or regain independence is important. Carers can help or hinder the older person who wishes to retain independence. The carer who 'takes over' and offers or insists on doing things for the person who can do it themselves is not helping and making things easier for the person. The carer is making life more difficult. Faced with such 'help' some older people can feel that there is little point in trying and that it is better to let the staff 'get on with it'.

Carers can unintentionally make older people feel useless. If a carer offers to bring a patient downstairs in a wheelchairs 'because it's quicker', the patient may soon lose the confidence and strength to come down alone. She will also lose independence and may begin to feel that she is a nuisance and a burden to staff. The sensitive carer will provide support and help without robbing the patient of her independence.

Mrs Edna Brown has lived in a nursing home for some time. At the morning report staff are informed that she fell whilst walking to bed the night before. The care assistant caring for her, Sarah Easton, asks Mrs Brown how she feels. Mrs Brown confesses that she feels shaken by her fall. Sarah offers to help her get her clothes ready and asks if she would like any help with washing or dressing. Mrs Brown says she can manage. Later Sarah walks with Mrs Brown to the lounge. This action gives Mrs Brown confidence; help is at hand if needed but Mrs Brown has maintained her independence.

Walking aids

Many older people rely on walking aids to help them move around. Some older people are admitted to homes with aids. Some individuals who do not have aids may be able to move around independently or with less help if they had an aid. There are several different types of walking aid. The commonest is the zimmer or walking frame.

Zimmer frames
Zimmer frames (Fig. 8.8a) help older people who are unsteady on their feet or who lack confidence, because when used properly people are more stable. Zimmer frames come in a variety of

(a)   (b)

Fig. 8.8   (a) Zimmer frame; (b) wheeled Zimmer frame.

heights and widths; it is possible to adjust the height on some frames. Each person is measured for their frame so that it is the right height. Too tall a frame encourages an individual to reach up; this unbalances the person and can cause falls. Too low a frame can lead to a person bending over the frame, which can also cause falls. When an older person has been measured for a frame it is important to label the frame so that frames don't become mixed up. This is an important safety measure if falls are to be prevented.

Zimmer frames have small rubber ends on each of the four legs, called ferrules. Each ferrule should have a whorl like pattern on it. These patterns of raised rubber prevent the frame from slipping. Carers should check every few months that the patterns have not worn off as worn ferrules can lead to the frame slipping and the individual falling. Ferrules can be replaced if this happens, new ones being obtained from the community supplies department of the local NHS trust.

Some older people, especially those suffering from arthritis, do not have the strength to lift a frame off the ground and are unable to use Zimmer frames. They are often supplied with special zimmer frames which have wheels at the bottom (Fig. 8.8b). The individual pushes the wheeled frame along. Wheeled frames are normally supplied after a careful assessment. An older person who tends to move quickly could easily fall or injure themselves using a wheeled frame. The wheels of these frames require oiling from time to time.

Gutter frames
Gutter frames are specialist frames. They are often supplied to individuals who have difficulty in gripping and lifting a normal frame (Fig. 8.9). Such frames are often supplied to individuals who have severe arthritis in the arms and hands. Such individuals may require the carer's help to stand up and gain their balance on the gutter frame. In many cases the carer will walk alongside the individual.

Tripods
Tripods are often used as walking aids by individuals who have suffered from strokes. The stroke may have left the individual with a weakness or paralysis on one side, which means that using a zimmer frame is not possible. Tripods should be fitted to ensure that they are the correct height. A person with a left sided weakness will require a right handed tripod and one with a right sided weakness a left handed tripod. Using a tripod allows the individual to improve balance and regain as much independence as possible. Sometimes people are able to walk alone using a tripod after a stroke; sometimes they need someone to help (Fig. 8.10).

Walking sticks
When older people feel unsteady they often buy walking sticks. It is important that walking sticks are the correct height for the individual and do not encourage stretching or stooping, which can lead to falls. Unfortunately few older people are measured for walking sticks. If an individual enters the home with walking sticks and these appear to be the wrong height, the height should be checked. Further details are given later in the chapter.

How aids are obtained

Many older people enter homes with aids. These may have been supplied in hospital or at home. The carer may feel that an older person might benefit from a walking aid. Sometimes an older

Fig. 8.9 Gutter frame.

person is no longer able to manage with a particular aid. The patient who managed well with a zimmer frame but who has suffered a stroke is no longer able to use her frame. She may benefit from a tripod.

Walking aids are normally supplied by the community physiotherapist. The procedure for obtaining aids varies from area to area. Normally the patient's doctor asks the physiotherapist to see the patient and assess for a walking aid. In some areas doctors are provided with special forms which they must complete, in others the doctor writes a letter to the physiotherapist. The physiotherapist visits and assesses the patient, then normally completes a form and orders the walking aid.

Fig. 8.10   Care Assistant helping an individual to use a tripod.

Walking aids are usually delivered direct to the home. Staff are often asked to call the physiotherapist when the aid arrives. The physiotherapist normally visits, makes any adjustments which are required and checks that the aid is safe and suitable.

Helping and encouraging older people to use their aids

Many patients are nervous when they first receive aids. Carers can help them gain confidence by encouraging them to use the aids. Older people who are getting used to using an aid should be accompanied on walks until staff are sure that they can walk safely and confidently alone. Some older people who use aids will always require someone to assist them. The use of an aid in such circumstances means that the older person can walk with an aid and one carer instead of two.

People who depend on aids should always have these placed near them. It is easy for a carer to move an aid out of the way when settling someone in bed and forget to place it back within reach of the individual before leaving the room. If someone is unable to reach their walking aid they may try to get up and walk without it. This can lead to a fall and the older person could suffer from a serious injury.

Using aids enables many older people to become more independent than before. Older people who use aids benefit from the exercise involved in walking. They feel more in control and are less likely to feel depressed. Family and friends may feel more confident about taking the individual on short outings and the individual's quality of life improves. The exercise improves the circulation to the legs and reduces the risk of swollen ankles and legs. Movement helps the bowel to work properly and the individual is less likely to become constipated. Gentle exercise such as walking may give patients who had no interest in food an appetite. Overweight patients benefit from exercise, and the ability to move around and go on outings will help them to lose weight. Staff within the home have more time to spend chatting or taking part in activities with the patient as they no longer have to spend so much time helping the person move around.

Wheelchairs

Helping people in wheelchairs retain and regain independence

Some people, because of disability or disease, are unable to walk even with aids and must use wheelchairs to help them move around. Patients with diseases such as multiple sclerosis or severe arthritis may need wheelchairs. People who are unable to walk can still retain independence if they are helped and encouraged to do so. Unfortunately many people are issued with wheelchairs which they cannot use themselves and they must rely on others to push them. This is a great shame as many people are able to learn how to move around in their wheelchairs. There are two different types of (non-electric) wheelchairs.

Self-propelling wheelchairs (Fig. 8.11) have large wheels which have circular metal hand grips around them. The older person uses the hand grip to turn the wheel and push herself along. Many people are able to become independent when they get used to their wheelchairs. Some people who have suffered from strokes have only one working hand with which to push the wheelchair. Stroke patients often request that the foot plate on the side of the body not affected by the stroke is left off. The patient then uses the unaffected leg to help steer and move the wheelchair around.

Fig. 8.11 Self-propelling wheelchair.

Other wheelchairs are designed for people who are unable to move around themselves (Fig. 8.12). These chairs have smaller wheels.

Transferring

Many older people can be encouraged and helped to move around the home in wheelchairs. Although the older person has lost the ability to walk, she has retained independence and is not forced to rely on carers to move around. Pushing a wheelchair around is fairly hard work and this exercise strengthens the muscles in the arms and chest. Many people who use wheelchairs can use these strong arm and chest muscles to transfer from wheelchair to chair, wheelchair to toilet or wheelchair to bed.

When transferring, the side of the wheelchair is normally removed. In some cases the individual is able to put some weight

Fig. 8.12   Non-self-propelling wheelchair.

on their legs and slide into a chair whilst holding onto one side of the wheelchair and the arm of the chair. When transferring from wheelchair to toilet, grab rails can be used to pull the body up. The carer can, if required, pull down clothing. The person can then use the grab rails to pull over and onto the toilet seat.

When transferring from bed to chair some patients use a special pole known as a 'monkey pole', which has a grip suspended from a chain. This grip helps the patient to lift up and swing over into the chair. Using a monkey pole requires strong muscles and the ability to lift the arms above the head. Some patients, especially those suffering from arthritis, are unable to use monkey poles. They may find using a special board (known as a transfer board) easier. One end of the board is placed on the wheelchair and the other on the bed (usually this end is placed under the mattress). The carer remains with the patient who uses the arms and, if possible, muscles in the lower body to wiggle along the board and into the bed or chair. The carer then removes the board.

Keeping wheelchairs in good repair

Older people who rely on wheelchairs to move around need chairs which are kept in good repair. Poorly maintained wheelchairs are at best difficult to use and at worst dangerous. Tyres should be kept firm. It is very difficult to push a wheelchair with flat tyres, and flat tyres can prevent wheelchair brakes from working properly. Wheelchairs which move when someone is transferring can cause falls. All wheelchairs are supplied with a pump and tyres which are becoming soft should be pumped up. You should find out who is responsible for this in your home. The home may employ maintenance staff or it may be the job of carers. Tyres which become soft again shortly after being pumped up may have a puncture. Wheelchair tyres should have a clearly visible tread on them. If the tread has worn away the tyres may need replacing.

Wheelchair brakes can easily become damaged; if the brakes are not working, urgent repairs should be organized.

Organizing repairs

Wheelchairs are supplied to individuals. Each wheelchair should have the individual's name on it. When wheelchairs are supplied to individuals in homes the manager is supplied with a reference number for each chair.

Arrangements for repair of wheelchairs vary from area to area. In some areas the community health trust (which is responsible for supplying and maintaining the wheelchairs of people living in homes) employs its own staff to repair wheelchairs. In other areas the community health trust employs a contractor to carry out repairs. The manager of your home will be able to tell you what the local arrangements are.

In all cases the staff responsible for carrying out repairs are telephoned. Often a message has to be left on an answerphone as staff are out repairing, collecting or delivering wheelchairs. The name of the patient, type of wheelchair and reference number, and if possible details of the fault, are required. The repairer requires these details so that spare parts which may be required can be brought along. If possible the chair will be repaired or parts such as tyres replaced at the home. If this is not possible the chair is taken away for repairs and a replacement chair is loaned to the patient until the wheelchair can be returned.

Exercise and passive movement

Carers should encourage patients to exercise and to move their limbs. Sometimes, though, patients are unable to do so. A patient who has lost all movement and feeling in the legs because of a disease such as multiple sclerosis will not be able to move her legs. A patient who has suffered from a severe stroke may be unable to understand or remember the carer's advice on moving his paralysed hand.

Joints which are not moved quickly stiffen up. The tendons, which connect joints, contract and shorten. Muscles become smaller and waste away. If the legs of an older person who is unable to move them are not moved, they can become fixed. A patient who sits for most of the day in a wheelchair can develop legs which are fixed in a permanent sitting position. If the legs are not gently moved and exercised by the carer it will become impossible to straighten them within a few months. These changes are known as flexion contractures. Carers can prevent such deformities by gently moving limbs which the patient is unable to move for themselves. If there is any existing deformity or limbs do not move normally carers should not attempt to move the limbs. A qualified nurse or doctor should be consulted.

Sometimes patients who have suffered from strokes are supplied with special aids, known as splints, to prevent deformities and contractures to the hand on the affected side. Splints and exercise or passive movement are used together. The splint prevents the hand from remaining in a closed position when it is not being exercised. If a patient has a splint, it is important to help put it on and encourage its use. There are several different types of hand splint. Each splint is made especially for the individual patient. A qualified nurse will be able to show you how splints are worn.

Summary

The aim of care is to help patients care for themselves as much as possible. Many older people admitted to homes have difficulty in moving around. The carer's approach and attitudes are vitally important in helping older people remain as independent as possible.

A carer's role is to support older people and help to retain independence. Many older people rely on aids to move around. Some people use wheelchairs but wheelchair users can still retain independence and freedom. Some people require assistance to move paralysed limbs to prevent deformity developing. Older people living within the home have an enormous range of abilities and carers who understand individual needs can work as part of the team to meet those needs.

Portfolio preparation

- Obtain information from the sources given in this chapter on how illness affects the ability to remain mobile.
- You may wish to visit a stroke club and see how these help people to recover after strokes.
- Find out what facilities are available locally to help people in homes make a full recovery after illness; for example, community physiotherapy or treatment at a day hospital.
- Outline ways in which your home encourages older people to remain mobile.
- Ask if you can copy a care plan showing how care for an individual is organized to encourage mobility and independence. Remember to remove the person's name from your copy to maintain confidentiality.

Chapter 9

Moving and Handling

Introduction

This chapter will give details of the legislation and policies relating to lifting and handling. It will outline:

- legal issues, including the Health & Safety at Work Act and The Manual Handling Regulations
- employer responsibilities
- employee responsibilities
- how great is the risk of back injury
- patient handling policies
- use of hoists and slings
- principles of safe lifting
- information on turning and lifting

This chapter gives the carer basic information on the principles of lifting and is intended to supplement practical workplace-based teaching of lifting methods.

Legal issues

The Health & Safety at Work Act (1974) outlined the responsibilities of employers to provide a safe working environment for staff. Further details are given in Chapter 6. The Manual Handling Regulations (1992) set out the maximum amount of weight each person could lift. They state that one person can lift a maximum of 25 kg and two can lift a maximum of 50 kg. People vary in the weights they can lift as some people are taller, heavier and stronger than others. Research indicates that the average female can only lift 16 kg safely. People's ability to lift varies. If a person is tired or feels unwell this affects the ability to lift. These regulations were introduced to reduce the incidence of back injury, not only in care settings but also in industry. The European Community Manual Handling of Loads Directive was introduced in December 1993.

Responsibilities of the employer

Employers are now obliged to take the following steps to reduce the incidence of back injury among staff:

- assess all manual handling tasks
- eliminate manual handling wherever possible
- reduce the risk of injury where there is no alternative to lifting
- ensure that staff are physically capable of lifting – pregnant staff and staff who have had a baby within the last three months should be assessed separately from other staff
- ensure that all staff receive training in lifting and handling
- ensure that equipment is provided
- monitor all accidents and sickness – take action to prevent accidents recurring wherever possible

The legislation obliges employers to provide equipment to enable staff to move patients safely. If people weigh more than 50 kg and are unable to move, staff will be required to use hoists to move them. The employer has a duty to provide equipment such as patient handling slings, transfer boards and hoists to enable staff to move patients safely, avoiding the risk of injury to either patients or staff.

Pregnant staff

Staff who are pregnant are less capable of lifting. In pregnancy the ligaments supporting the spine loosen and the pregnant member of staff is at greater risk of back injury than any other member of staff. In most homes there is a policy that pregnant staff do not lift, as this would be detrimental to their health and the health of those whom they care for. In some small homes it is not possible to have a member of staff on duty who is not able to lift. In these circumstances the employer has a duty to find alternative work (at the same rate of pay) for the pregnant employee.

The employee has a duty to inform the employer as soon as she is aware of her pregnancy, so that steps can be taken to reduce the risk of injury to the member of staff, to other staff members (if the employee is unable to lift safely) and to patients.

Employee responsibilities

Employees have a duty under the legislation to take reasonable care of their own health and safety and those who may be affected by their omissions, and to co-operate with the employer. This means that employees:

- have a duty to attend training sessions
- should comply with lifting policies within the home
- should not use lifts which have proved to be dangerous
- should use equipment provided
- should report any faults in equipment promptly
- should remove dangerous equipment from use.

The Health & Safety Executive

If it is 'reasonably practical' for the employer to comply with legal requirements and they fail to do so, the Health & Safety Executive can take action; for example, if a hoist is required to help heavily dependent patients bathe and the bathroom will accommodate a hoist but the employer fails to provide one. The Health & Safety Executive employs health and safety inspectors who visit and serve a notice obliging the employer to supply equipment. The inspector specifies a period of time in which the employer must comply. The inspector will then return to ensure that the equipment has been supplied. If the employer fails to comply he or she may be prosecuted under section 2(2) a–e of the Health & Safety at Work Act 1974. Employers who fail to comply can be imprisoned for up to two years and face unlimited fines.

How great is the risk of back injury?

Staff working with elderly people are at greater risk of injuring their backs than staff working with other client groups. Backs can be injured not only by using unsafe lifts or by accidents, they can also be injured by the strain of lifting day in and day out for years. Research has shown that in some areas of nursing such as elderly care a nurse can lift a ton in the course of a shift.

Staff working with the elderly are more likely to suffer from backpain as a result of lifting. One survey discovered that 28% of nurses working on surgical wards in NHS hospitals suffered from backpain at least once a week. In elderly care wards 92% of staff suffered from regular backpain.

Uniforms can increase the risk of back injury. In the UK staff normally wear dresses with narrow skirts. These restrict movement and make it more difficult to lift properly and avoid the risk of injury. In other countries such as the United States and Australia research has shown that nurses who wear tunics and trousers are much less likely to suffer from back injury (Fig. 9.1).

Staff working with elderly people can, with the best of intentions, lift and handle older people who with aids, instruction and

Fig. 9.1 Uniforms such as these reduce the risk of back injury because movement is unrestricted.

encouragement could move themselves. This practice causes the older person to become more dependent on staff and increases staff workload.

Patient handling policies

Homes should now carry out an assessment of any person who requires help to move. In many homes a standard assessment form has been drafted. This form should be simple and easy to fill in; an example is given in Fig. 9.2.

In nursing homes the assessment should be carried out by a registered nurse. In residential homes assessments will be carried out either by the manager or a senior member of staff. If staff in homes require further advice they can contact the community physiotherapist for the area.

The information from the assessment is used to draw up a plan of care which is referred to when handling the patient. The care plan should specify:

■ the equipment required to move the person – this may be a sling, hoist, frame or monkey pole
■ the number of staff required to carry out a handling procedure
■ what the patient can do to help
■ any other information which staff require

Handling assessment form

Name:_____

Weight:_____

Body shape:

       Tall _____   Short _____ Medium _____

       Obese _____ Thin _____ Average _____

Patients comprehension/ability to co-operate:_____

_____

Behaviour which may affect lifting/handling:_____

_____

Disability/weakness/deformity:_____

_____

Handling constraints:_____

  Pain:_____

  Skin type:_____

  Other:_____

Difficulties and solutions:_____

  Walking:_____

  Standing:_____

  Toileting:_____

  To/from bed:_____

  Movement in bed:_____

  Equipment normally used:_____

Methods of moving: manual/hoist:_____

Assessed by:_____   Date:_____

Fig. 9.2 Patient handling assessment.

Date	Needs	Aim	Action	Evaluation
23/6/95	To help	1) To lift her	1) Use shoulder lift	1) Shoulder
	Mrs Jones	up in bed	(Mrs Jones weighs	lift
	sit comfortably	maintaining	47 kg and has no pain	effective.
	in bed.	patient	or history of shoulder	
		comfort and	injury).	
		staff safety		
		2) To lift		
	Is having	Mrs Jones		
	difficulty sitting	clear of bed		
	up and moving	without		
	up in bed, due	dragging.		
	to an acute	3) To prevent		
	attack of	skin damage		
	bronchitis.	caused by		
		dragging.		

Name: Room No: Age:

Fig. 9.3   Care plan for lifting.

An example of a care plan is given in Fig. 9.3. Care plans should be reviewed regularly and if the person's abilities change and the methods of handling change these must be noted on the care plan.

Training

All staff should receive training before lifting. Carers should not lift until they have been trained to do so. Staff should receive regular updating on lifting and handling skills.

Using hoists

If a person weighs more than 50 kg and is unable to assist in moving, staff should use a hoist. Many homes have hoists, together with policies which state that staff should use these to move patients weighing more than 50 kg, yet staff continue to lift patients manually, risking the health of the patient, their colleagues and themselves. Research has shown that there are a number of reasons why staff do not use hoists, including:

- insufficient room to move the hoist around
- the hoist will not fit in the toilet or bathroom
- the hoist is poorly maintained – the wheels may stick or staff may struggle to use it
- staff have not been trained to use the hoist
- the patient dislikes the hoist
- other staff do not use the hoist

Hoists are used to move patients. The patient is held in a sling which is attached to the hoist, enabling staff to raise, move and lower the patient (Fig. 9.4). There are a number of different hoists on the market; each comes with an instruction booklet.

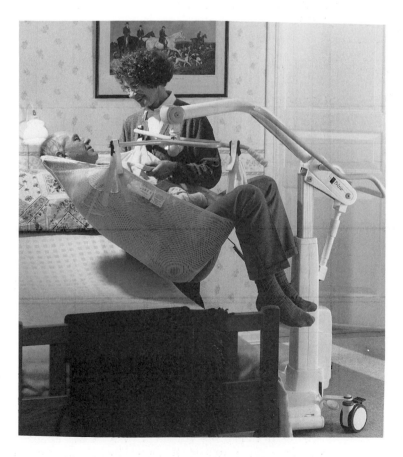

Fig. 9.4 A Trixie hoist.

Slings

Each hoist manufacturer makes several different slings for use with their hoist. Carers should never use the sling from one manufacturer with the hoist made by another as they may not fit properly and can cause accidents.

Some slings consist of two pieces. One part of the sling slips behind the patient's back and under the arms; the other is placed under the patient's thighs and both are attached to the hoist. Department of Health guidance has been issued instructing homes not to use two part slings for elderly people as several serious accidents have occurred involving their use.

Principles of safe lifting

Although staff use a number of different lifting techniques to move patients, the same basic principles should be used at all times:

- Ensure that you have enough space in which to lift. Move furniture and equipment if necessary. If the person requires help to move you may find it easier to rearrange the furniture in the room. If the bed is against the wall and two staff are required to move the person, it makes sense to re-arrange the furniture so that staff have access to both sides of the bed.
- Never lift a patient if the patient can move without lifting, or the patient is at risk of becoming physically weaker and losing the ability to move independently. You unnecessarily place yourself at risk of injury.
- Assess the patient and decide what method of lifting is required.
- Ensure that you have enough people or the correct equipment to move the person.
- Explain to the patient what you intend to do. Ask the patient to co-operate. Explain what you wish the patient to do. Check that the patient has understood.
- Be aware of your ability and that of your lifting partner.
- Keep your feet apart; make sure you are balanced.
- Lift towards yourself, *never* away from you.
- Hold the patient as close to you as possible.
- Do not twist your body when lifting.
- Raise your head as you lift. This helps keep your back straight and reduces the risk of injury.
- When lifting with a partner check that you are both clear about the type of lift you are using and what you will both be doing. Use a signal so that you both lift together; for example one, two, three, lift; or ready, steady, lift.

Turning patients in bed

People who cannot turn over in bed without help are at risk of developing pressure sores. Details on preventing pressure sores are given in Chapter 10. If the person is unable to turn over, staff must turn the person.

Staff can use a strong draw sheet with a plastic backing, to help turn the patient. It is very important that you check that the draw sheet is strong and in good condition before using it. A nurse who used a worn draw sheet to turn a patient, and the draw sheet ripped, suffered a serious back injury. In this case because staff had reported that the draw sheets were worn and the employer had not replaced them, the nurse was awarded damages. The judge, commenting on the case, stated that he would not have awarded damages had staff not previously reported the condition of the draw sheets.

- assess the task
- if the person is very heavy two members of staff may be required to roll the patient, whilst a third prevents the person from rolling off the bed
- roll the patient onto his back
- use the drawsheet to move him to the side of the bed
- a draw sheet with a plastic undersheet helps the patient to slide more easily and prevents friction (also known as shearing forces) from damaging the patient's skin and increasing the risk of pressure sores developing
- move the patient's head and shoulders
- move the patient's legs
- move the patient's trunk
- the second nurse (or third if two are required to roll the patient) is at the opposite side of the bed and prevents the patient from rolling out of bed

The shoulder lift

This lift (Fig. 9.5) may also be referred to as the Australian lift. It is useful for sitting patients up in bed and transferring patients from bed to chair. It is not suitable for all patients and should not be used if:

- the person can move herself
- the patient weighs more than 50 kg
- the patient has any injury, disease or pain in the shoulder – for example if they are suffering from weakness or paralysis on one side following a stroke, have difficulty in moving the

shoulder perhaps because of pain or stiffness, or have arthritis of the shoulder
- the patient has pain or injury affecting the chest or the upper part of the back
- the patient has had recent hip surgery
- the patient is confused and unable to co-operate with staff

This lift enables staff to lift the person effectively and reduce stress

Fig. 9.5   Shoulder lift.

to their backs. It lifts the patient clear of the bed and reduces the risk of friction contributing to the development of pressure sores. To carry out the lift:

- one carer stands at each side of the bed
- sit the patient forward
- one carer supports the patient
- the other adjusts the pillows
- both carers place their near shoulders into the patient's chest wall just below the armpit (axilla)
- the patient puts his arms down the carer's backs
- carers place their near arms under the patient's thighs as close to the buttocks as possible
- carers use a wrist or finger grip to hold each other's hands
- place the other hand on the bed behind the patient
- place near knee on the bed
- lift together on the agreed signal

The two sling lift

The two sling lift (Fig. 9.6) can also be used to lift a patient up in bed, but there is a risk of dragging the patient's heels with this lift. If the patient's heels are red or are judged to be at risk of developing pressure sores, they must be protected before this lift is carried out. Make sure that the person has heel protectors on and that these are in the correct position.

This lift should only be carried out if the person weighs less than 50 kg. Two members of staff are required

- staff face each other from opposite sides of the bed
- place one patient handling sling under the patient's buttocks and upper thighs
- place the second sling under the lower back, upper waist
- place your near knee on the bed
- grip one end of each sling
- lift together on the agreed signal

Summary

It is now recommended that carers lift people only as a last resort. Whenever possible the emphasis should be on teaching, helping and encouraging people to move themselves. All homes where people require lifting should provide suitable equipment to enable patients to be moved without either patient or carer risking injury. The aim of this chapter is to provide an introduction to lifting

(a)

(b)

(c)

Fig. 9.6 The three stages involved in using a two sling lift: (a) position the sling beneath the patient's thighs; (b) raise the patient to the upright, sitting position; (c) position the second sling behind the patient's back and ensure it fits comfortably under their arms.

practice. It is important that you receive training before moving patients.

Portfolio preparation

■ Collect details on the lifting and handling policy in your home.
■ Include a blank copy of a patient assessment sheet.
■ You may wish to ask the matron or manager of the home for permission to copy information from a care plan relating to lifting and handling. Remember not to use the person's name, so as to maintain confidentiality of patient information. You may wish to use a false name or the person's initials.
■ Collect details of training which you have undertaken in the home.

Further reading

Hollis, M. (1991) *Safer Lifting for Patient Care.* Blackwell Science, Oxford.

National Backpain Association (1992) *The Guide to the Handling of Patients*, 3rd edn. National Backpain Association, Teddington, Middlesex.

Health and Safety Executive (1992) *Management of Health & Safety at Work.* HMSO, London.

Health & Safety Executive (1992) *Manual Handling Guidance on Regulations, L22.* HMSO, London.

Health and Safety Commission (1992) *Management of Health & Safety at Work. Approved Code of Practice.* HMSO, London.

Management of Health and Safety at Work Regulations (1992) *Statutory Instrument no 2051.* HMSO, London.

Chapter 10

Preventing Pressure Sores

Introduction

Most pressure sores can be prevented. The development of a pressure sore, in most cases, is a sign that care is not of a high standard and that staff failed to take action to prevent the sore developing. Staff who understand why pressure sores develop can take action to prevent them occurring. This chapter gives information on:

- how pressure sores develop
- treating pressure sores
- where pressure sores develop
- which patients are most at risk and why
- assessing risk
- the principles of preventing pressure sores
- using aids such as beds, mattresses, cushions, heel and elbow protectors
- caring for the whole person

Pressure sores

Pressure sores are commonly called bedsores. Doctors and nurses often refer to them by the technical name of *decubitus ulcers.* They will be referred to throughout this chapter as pressure sores.

Pressure sores are caused by pressure, friction or shearing forces applied to the skin. A person does not have to be confined to bed to develop pressure sores. Many people who are sitting in chairs all day are in danger of developing pressure sores. Pressure sores are areas of skin which have been damaged by unrelieved pressure, friction or shearing forces or a combination of these three factors.

How pressure sores develop

Pressure sores develop when a part of the body is not moved. Normally the skin is nourished by small blood vessels called *capillaries*. Capillaries carry blood which delivers oxygen and glucose to the skin. If blood supply to the skin is cut off, the skin and deeper tissues die. Unrelieved pressure on any area of the body interrupts the capillary blood flow and can lead to tissue death. Poor lifting and moving techniques, which drag rather than lift, are known as *shearing forces.* This can cause tissue damage which leads to the development of pressure sores.

Normally when a patient begins to develop a pressure sore the first sign is a red mark on the skin. If you place a finger lightly on the red area and it whitens this shows that the capillary circulation is undamaged. With care the patient may avoid developing a pressure sore. If the skin remains red when light finger pressure is applied, capillary circulation has been damaged. There may be a slight sore or blister on the skin.

At one time it was recommended that reddened skin was massaged. It was thought that a firm massage improved the circulation and got the blood flowing back into the reddened skin. However, researchers found that massaging reddened skin did not improve circulation and actually caused further damage and made it more likely that the patient would develop pressure sores. *Reddened skin should not under any circumstances be massaged.*

Pressure sore gradings

If action is not taken to relieve pressure regularly, areas of reddened skin can quickly develop into serious pressure sores. There are five stages of pressure sores:

(1) skin reddening which whitens when you press a finger lightly on the skin
(2) skin reddening which remains red when you press a finger lightly on the skin
(3) skin ulcers
(4) deeper ulcer where the fat beneath the skin is also ulcerated; the muscle underneath is swollen
(5) deep ulcers where skin, fat, muscle and sometimes bone are damaged by pressure.

Pressure sore sites

Pressure sores can develop on any part of the body (Fig. 10.1). They can occur on ears, cheeks, arms, trunk, legs and heels. Most pressure sores develop between the buttocks on the bony area known as the sacrum. A patient lying on a hard mattress for a few hours can develop a pressure sore if she is unable to move and is not moved by carers. Patients sitting in chairs also develop sacral pressure sores.

The heels are also a common site for pressure sores. A patient who is sitting with his heels up on a footstool is just as much at risk as the patient whose heels are resting on a mattress in bed.

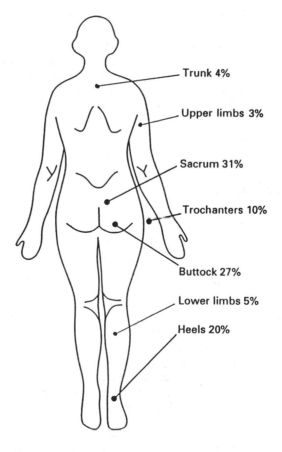

Trunk 4%

Upper limbs 3%

Sacrum 31%

Trochanters 10%

Buttock 27%

Lower limbs 5%

Heels 20%

Fig. 10.1   Common sites of pressure sores.

Which patients are at risk of developing pressure sores?

Older people are 20 times more likely to develop pressure sores than people in their twenties and thirties. Women are more likely to develop pressure sores than men, because women have a higher proportion of body fat than men. Fat has poorer blood supply than muscle or lean tissue. People who suffer from a long standing illness are more likely to develop pressure sores than people in good health. Most older people living in homes have been admitted because of poor health and therefore are at greater risk of developing pressure sores than people who live in their own homes.

Confused patients
Confused patients are at risk of developing pressure sores. Many confused patients sit quietly for hours and staff may be busy attending to more alert patients who are able to ask for help. The confused person may not be aware of the discomfort or pain caused by remaining in one position for a long time. Sometimes the patient is aware of the discomfort but is unable to tell carers what the problem is. Some confused patients are prescribed sedatives because they become agitated. Sedatives can make older people drowsy and less aware. Patients who are drowsy will be less aware of pain and discomfort.

Patients who cannot move or walk around without help
Normally people who are able to move around will feel stiff and uncomfortable if they are sitting or lying in one position. Getting up and walking or rolling over in bed will relieve pressure and prevent tissue damage. Patients who are unable to move around without help rely on carers to help them turn over, get up or change position. If an older person at high risk of developing pressure sores is not moved or helped to move, severe skin damage can occur and a deep pressure sore can develop.

People who are paralysed
Patients who have suffered from strokes may be paralysed down one side of the body. They may not be able to feel anything on the paralysed side and may be unaware of discomfort and pressure. They may also be unable to move without help. Some stroke patients may have difficulty in communicating with carers and asking for help when they feel uncomfortable.

Patients who suffer from diseases of the brain (referred to as neurological diseases), such as multiple sclerosis or motor neurone disease, may lose all sensation in the lower part of the body. As the disease advances patients may have difficulty in moving and speaking.

People with heart disease and high blood pressure
People with heart disease and high blood pressure are at risk of developing pressure sores because they have poor circulation. People with poor circulation develop pressure sores more quickly than people with normal circulation.

People with diabetes
People with diabetes often suffer from poor circulation. Patients with mild diabetes, which is treated with a special diet, are less at risk than diabetics who require tablets to help control diabetes. Patients who require insulin injections to control diabetes are more likely to suffer from poor circulation than other diabetics.

Some diabetic patients, especially those who require insulin injections, develop loss of feeling in the feet, lower parts of the legs and the hands. This condition is known as *peripheral neuropathy*, and there is no treatment for it. Diabetic patients are at great risk of developing pressure sores on the heels as they are often unaware of pain or discomfort caused by pressure. Poor circulation and the effects of diabetes, which slow down the rate of wound healing, make it difficult to heal such pressure sores if they develop.

People who are overweight or underweight
These people are more likely to develop pressure sores. Overweight people have poorer circulation than people of normal weight. Many overweight people have a poor diet which is too high in sugars and low in vitamins. A diet low in vitamins affects the health of the skin and increases the risk of pressure sores.

Underweight people are even more likely than overweight people to develop pressure sores. Thin people lack a layer of fat which protects muscle from the effects of pressure, and thin people are much more at risk of the effects of shearing forces because their bones are more prominent.

People who are incontinent
People who are incontinent of faeces and urine are at greater risk of developing pressure sores than those who are incontinent of urine only. Incontinent patients can develop skin rashes if pads are not changed frequently or if the skin is not carefully washed after each episode of incontinence. Patients who are incontinent of faeces may wet on a soiled pad. This causes the release of ammonia and can cause skin to become sore and red very quickly.

Skin soreness and rashes cause the skin to become inflamed. Sore, inflamed skin can develop blisters and boils. These can become infected. People who have sore or infected skin are more at risk of developing pressure sores than people who have healthy skin.

Many people who are incontinent wear pads. If pads are not put on properly, ridges from the pad can cause pressure on the skin and this can lead to pressure sores. There are many different types of pad. The quality of pad varies, as does the cost. All pads are made of paper (cellulose) pulp. This is covered by a one way liner which is designed to draw urine away from the patient's skin and into the pad. Most pads have a plastic backing to prevent urine leaking onto the patient's clothes. Some pads contain more pulp than others. Some pads also contain super absorbent crystals. The crystals turn into a gel and lock urine into the pad. Pads which contain more cellulose pulp and super absorbent crystals keep the skin of incontinent patients drier between changes. Skin which is dry is less likely to become sore, infected or develop pressure sores.

The effects of pressure sores

Pressure sores can cause a great deal of pain and discomfort. Pain can prevent an older person moving around, chatting and taking part in the activities of the home, and can prevent the older person from getting a good night's sleep. Doctors can prescribe pain killers, and people with large or deep pressure sores may require strong pain killers. Unfortunately strong pain killers can make some patients feel sick and can cause constipation. Lack of sleep can make the individual feel unwell.

Pressure sores, especially those on the sacrum and the hips, can easily become infected and infection can cause the patient to develop a high temperature and to feel unwell. The patient may feel too unwell to eat, yet a diet full of protein, vitamins and carbohydrates is essential if the wound is to heal.

Patients who have infected wounds are usually prescribed antibiotics by their doctors. Antibiotics can make some patients feel sick and lose their appetites. Some patients can also suffer from diarrhoea when prescribed antibiotics.

Infected wounds often smell. Some wounds, because of the bacteria with which they are infected, smell dreadful. This can be very upsetting for the patient. Some patients who develop deep pressure sores can suffer from infection which infects the bone. They can develop blood poisoning (septicaemia) and even with hospital treatment some patients will not survive.

Patients who have developed pressure sores will require wound dressings. These will be carried out by registered nurses in nursing homes; in residential homes the district nurse will visit to carry out dressings. Many older people who have developed pressure sores become depressed. Some are so depressed that they feel life is not worth living and require antidepressant tablets.

How trained nurses assess who is at risk of developing pressure sores

Carers in nursing homes work under the direction of a trained nurse. Carers are often part of a team and are responsible for the care of a small group of patients, although of course they help care for all patients within the home. The trained nurse works with the patient and carers and decides what care is required. Trained nurses use specially designed charts which assess those patients who are at risk of developing pressure sores and how great the risk is. The nurse can then decide on a plan of care which all members of the team carry out.

There are several scales to assess risk but the two most commonly used by trained nurses are the *Norton scale* and the *Waterlow scale*.

The Norton scale (Fig. 10.2) was developed in 1962. It assesses the patient's general health, mental state, activity, mobility and continence. Patients score points based on these categories. An individual in poor health, who is confused, immobile and incontinent, will have a lower score than an individual who is in poor health but who is alert, walks with help and is continent. The total points are added up and this is known as the Norton score. A score of 16 points or below indicates that the patient is at risk of

Physical condition	Mental state	Activity	Mobility	Incontinence
Good 4	Alert 4	Ambulant 4	Full 4	None 4
Fair 3	Apathetic 3	Walks with	Slightly	Occasional 3
Poor 2	Confused 2	help 3	limited 3	Usually
Very bad 1	Stuporous 1	Chairbound 2	Very	urinary 2
		Bedfast 1	limited 2	Double 1
			Immobile 1	

Patient total score:
Implications:

Fig. 10.2 Norton scale.

WATERLOW PRESSURE SORE PREVENTION/TREATMENT POLICY

RING SCORES IN TABLE, ADD TOTAL.   SEVERAL SCORES PER CATEGORY CAN BE USED

BUILD/WEIGHT FOR HEIGHT	★	SKIN TYPE VISUAL RISK AREAS	★	SEX AGE	★	SPECIAL RISKS	★
AVERAGE	0	HEALTHY	0	MALE	1	TISSUE MALNUTRITION	★
ABOVE AVERAGE	1	TISSUE PAPER	1	FEMALE	2		
OBESE	2	DRY	1	14 - 49	1	e.g.: TERMINAL CACHEXIA	8
BELOW AVERAGE	3	OEDEMATOUS	1	50 - 64	2	CARDIAC FAILURE	5
		CLAMMY (TEMP↑)	1	65 - 74	3	PERIPHERAL VASCULAR	
CONTINENCE	★	DISCOLOURED	2	75 - 80	4	DISEASE	5
		BROKEN/SPOT	3	81+	5	ANAEMIA	2
COMPLETE/						SMOKING	1
CATHETERISED	0	**MOBILITY**	★	**APPETITE**	★		
OCCASION INCONT	1					**NEUROLOGICAL DEFICIT**	★
CATH/INCONTINENT							
OF FAECES	2	FULLY	0	AVERAGE	0	eg: DIABETES, M.S, CVA,	
DOUBLY INCONT	3	RESTLESS/FIDGETY	1	POOR	1	MOTOR/SENSORY	
		APATHETIC	2	N.G. TUBE/		PARAPLEGIA	4 - 6
		RESTRICTED	3	FLUIDS ONLY	2		
		INERT/TRACTION	4	NBM/ANOREXIC	3	**MAJOR SURGERY/TRAUMA**	★
		CHAIRBOUND	5				
						ORTHOPAEDIC -	
						BELOW WAIST,SPINAL	5
						ON TABLE > 2 HOURS	5

SCORE	10+ AT RISK	15+ HIGH RISK	20+ VERY HIGH RISK

MEDICATION	★
CYTOTOXICS, HIGH DOSE STEROIDS ANTI-INFLAMMATORY	4

© J Waterlow 1991 Revised March 1992

OBTAINABLE FROM: NEWTONS, CURLAND, TAUNTON, TA3 5SG

REMEMBER: TISSUE DAMAGE OFTEN STARTS PRIOR TO ADMISSION, IN CASUALTY. A SEATED PATIENT IS ALSO AT RISK

ASSESSMENT: (See Over)   IF THE PATIENT FALLS INTO ANY OF THE RISK CATEGORIES THEN PREVENTATIVE NURSING IS REQUIRED.
A COMBINATION OF GOOD NURSING TECHNIQUES AND PREVENTATIVE AIDS WILL DEFINITELY BE NECESSARY.

PREVENTION:

PREVENTATIVE AIDS:

Special Mattress/ Bed:
10+Overlays or specialist foam mattresses
15+Alternating pressure overlays, mattresses and bed systems.
20+Bed Systems: Fluidised, bead, low air loss and alternating pressure mattresses.
Note: Preventative aids cover a wide spectrum of specialist features. Efficacy in the 20+ area should be judged on the basis of independent evidence.

Cushions:
No patient should sit in a wheelchair without some form of cushioning. If nothing else is available - use the patient's own pillow.
10+ 4" Foam cushion.
15+ Specialist Gell and/or foam cushion
20+ Cushion capable of adjustment to suit individual patient.

Bed Clothing:
Avoid plastic draw sheets, inco pads and tightly tucked in sheets/sheet covers, especially when using Specialist bed and mattress overlay systems.
Duvet - plus vapour permeable cover

NURSING CARE:

General: Frequent changes of position, lying or sitting.
Use of pillows?
Pain   Appropriate pain control
Nutrition   High Protein, vitamins, minerals
Patient Handling: Correct lifting technique
Hoists
Monkey Pole
Transfer devices
Patient Comfort Aids: Real sheepskins
Bed cradle
Operating Table/   4" cover plus adequate protection
Theatre/A&E Trolley
Skin Care: General Hygiene, NO rubbing.
Correct lifting and positioning.
Cover with an appropriate dressing

IF TREATMENT IS REQUIRED, FIRST REMOVE PRESSURE

WOUND CLASSIFICATION:

BLANCHING HYPERAEMIA	STAGE I	Is wound RED?	YES Semi-permeable film hydrocolloid sheet
NON-BLANCHING HYPERAEMIA	STAGE II	Is wound RED, clean but not healed?	YES Hydrocolloid, alginate, hydrogel, Silastic Foam (deep)
ULCERATION PROGRESSES	STAGE III	Is wound YELLOW/ infected/inflamed?	YES Alginate, hydrogel, hydrocolloid
ULCERATION EXTENDS	STAGE IV	Infected?	YES Alginate ribbon or rope, non adherent topical antimicrobial dressing, polysaccharide paste
INFECTIVE NECROSIS	STAGE V	Is wound BLACK/ Necrotic?	YES Debride-surgical excision, hydrocolloid, hydrogel, enzymatic treatment.

Fig. 10.3 Waterlow scale.

developing a pressure sore. The lower the score the higher the risk of the patient developing pressure sores.

The Waterlow scale (Fig. 10.3) was developed as a result of research carried out in 1985, and is a more detailed assessment scale. It assesses factors such as build, weight, continence, skin type, mobility, sex, age and appetite. The score has special high risk factors such as surgery, medication, age and diseases. Each risk factor carries points and the points are added up. A score of 10 indicates that the patient is at risk of developing pressure sores; a score of 15–20 indicates that the patient is at high risk and a score of more than 20 indicates that the patient is at very high risk. The higher the score the greater the risk of the patient developing pressure sores.

Using a scoring system enables qualified nurses to identify those patients who are at high risk and to plan care which will prevent pressure scores developing. Patients in nursing homes normally have a pressure sore risk assessment completed when they enter the home. People living in residential homes are usually more mobile and less at risk of pressure sores. They do not normally have a pressure sore risk assessment carried out unless carers notice that their skin is becoming red. Then carers normally contact the district nurse who will carry out an assessment.

People living in residential homes who are at very high risk of developing a pressure sore may require nursing home care. Residential homes must abide by the Registered Homes Act[1]. This Act states that people living in residential homes should receive the care which could be given at home by a caring relative. The older person at high risk of developing a pressure sore will require higher levels of care than most residential homes can provide. This is because residential homes have fewer staff, few employ trained nurses, and most do not have special aids which the individual may require.

When a pressure sore risk assessment has been carried out in a nursing home, the qualified nurse will note this in the care plan. The note should give the date of the assessment and the scale used. If the score indicates that the patient is at risk a plan of care will be written. This will give instructions on how care will be planned to prevent pressure sores.

In residential homes the district nurse will leave details of the patient's care in the patient's case notes. These are left in the home so that other district nurses who call are aware of treatment required. The district nurse will give carers instructions and carers should make a note of these instructions in the patient records.

Preventing pressure sores

Pressure sores are caused by unrelieved pressure which affects blood flow and causes sores to develop. Relieving the pressure and moving patients allows blood to flow normally to the tissues and prevents pressure sores developing. Patients who are sitting all day are just as much at risk of developing pressure sores as patients who are nursed in bed. Patients who are sitting in chairs and who are able to walk should be encouraged to do so. Encouraging and helping an older person to walk to the dining room for lunch will help prevent a pressure sore. Serving lunch on a tray may mean the individual continues to sit and pressure on the bottom is unrelieved.

Many patients are unable to walk without help. Carers should encourage patients to walk, walking with them and encouraging them to walk at their own pace. Offering to wheel the patient to the dining area does little to relieve pressure and help circulation. Patients who are unable to walk can be encouraged to stand. The patient can use a Zimmer frame, grab rails or be supported by staff. Encouraging patients to stand, even with help, not only helps prevent pressure sores but prevents joints becoming stiff and reduces the risk of the patient's legs developing deformities such as flexion contractures. Details of flexion contractures are given in Chapter 8. Patients who are unable to walk or stand are at risk of pressure sores and should not sit all day in the same chair as this will almost certainly cause pressure sores.

Older people require less sleep than younger people and tire more easily than when they were young. Older people are more likely to have a nap in the afternoon and often sleep for an hour after lunch. In many homes older people fall asleep in their chairs after lunch. They may awake feeling stiff, uncomfortable and not refreshed by their sleep.

Encouraging frail older people who feel tired to go to bed for a nap will help prevent pressure sores. Carers can assist the individual to bed and can help the person to lie on one side, which will relieve pressure on the bottom. The older person will sleep comfortably and awake refreshed ready for a cup of tea, a visit from family or friends or activities in the home.

People normally turn over in bed whilst asleep. Moving around in bed prevents us from developing pressure sores whilst we sleep. Many frail older people who are at risk of pressure sores are unable to turn over in bed. All patients who are at risk should be turned every two hours. The patient is normally nursed on his back for two hours, then turned onto perhaps the left side. Two hours later the patient is turned onto the right side. If a patient's sacrum is becoming red, they may lie on one hip and then the other, avoiding wherever possible any pressure on the sacrum. If one of the hips is becoming red, the patient may lie only on the other hip or on the sacrum. If a patient is lying on his or her side there is a risk that they will roll back onto the back. A soft pillow is often placed either under the mattress or at the back of the patient, to prevent this.

Mattresses and beds used to prevent pressure sores developing

Older people who are at risk of developing pressure sores may still develop pressure sores even if turned every two hours. It can be difficult to turn patients more frequently. Often two staff are needed to turn the patient. If two staff work together the patient is at less risk of shearing forces which can cause pressure sores, and carers reduce the risk of developing a back injury. Details on moving and handling patients are given in Chapter 9.

Patients who are turned every hour have little opportunity to rest or sleep. Many different types of mattresses and beds have been designed so that the risk of developing pressure sores is reduced. Pressure relieving equipment is available which either replaces the existing mattress or lies on top of the existing mattress.

Pressure relieving mattresses and overlays

These are designed to take the pressure away from the patient's skin at regular intervals (Fig. 10.4). They are normally made of horizontal cells of air which inflate and deflate on a cycle. This cycle is controlled by an electrical pump. The alternate cells which are inflated support the patient, whilst the deflated cells are relieving the pressure to that area of the patient's body. Alternating pressure mattresses/overlays are sometimes referred to as ripple mattresses. Pressure relieving mattresses are used for the prevention of pressure sores and also the treatment of any existing sores.

Some pressure relieving mattresses/overlays automatically adjust the amount of air in the cells. They are able to adjust to the weight and position of the patient. Others, however, have a small dial which needs to be set according to the weight of the patient. There is normally a printed table on the electronic pump giving details about which settings should be used for people within certain weight ranges.

Pressure relieving mattresses and overlays (Figs 10.5 and 10.6) are used for all levels of risk and grade of pressure sore. It is important that you seek advice from a trained nurse if you are unsure which product is suitable for an individual patient.

Fig. 10.4 Alternating pressure relieving mattress replacement. (Courtesy Huntleigh Healthcare.)

Most pressure relieving mattresses/overlays have a special vapour permeable multi-stretch cover. This vapour permeability allows the patient's skin to breathe and prevents the patient from becoming hot and sweaty. This means that the skin is less likely to become macerated. The covers are water resistant and the multi-stretch properties help to prevent the cover wrinkling and bunching up and reduce friction. Manufacturers recommend that the covers are washed with soap and water. Disinfectants, detergents and deodorisers should not be sprayed onto the covers. The covers should not be sent to the laundry as laundering will ruin them. If you are unsure ask a trained nurse who will check the manufacturer's cleaning guidance.

When using a pressure relieving mattress/overlay the sheet should not be tucked in tightly and Kylie-type bedsheets, draw sheets and incontinence pads should be avoided as they greatly reduce the effectiveness of pressure relieving mattresses. It is best to leave the pressure relieving mattress/overlay switched on even when not in use. The motor has to work harder to re-inflate than to maintain the inflated pressure. Deflating the mattress means that the patient cannot go back to bed if tired as the mattress/overlay should be inflated before the patient uses it.

Fig. 10.5   Alternating pressure relieving overlay.
(Courtesy Huntleigh Healthcare.)

Fig. 10.6   Silicore fibre overlay. (Courtesy Huntleigh Healthcare.)

Pressure reducing overlays and mattresses are often made of foam or fibre. These reduce pressure by moulding to the contours of the patient's body so that there is a greater surface area in contact with the overlay. This distributes the patient's weight more evenly and reduces the pressure.

Pressure reducing overlays and mattresses should only be used to *prevent* pressure sores. They are not suitable for patients who have developed pressure sores. These types of mattresses/overlays are normally used to help prevent pressure sores in patients who are at low to medium risk of developing them. It is important to seek advice from a trained nurse who can check the manufacturer's recommendations. These mattresses and overlays are available with vapour permeable covers.

In some nursing homes, hospices and in hospital very specialised beds such as low air loss (Fig. 10.7) and fluidised bead beds are sometimes used for patients who are very ill, have existing pressure sores and cannot easily be moved. If you require any further information on these specialised beds, ask a qualified member of staff.

Fig. 10.7 Low airloss bed. (Courtesy KCI Mediscus.)

Cushions and pressure relieving aids

People who are at risk of developing pressure sores are at even greater risk when they are sitting in chairs. A range of cushions should be available within the home to help prevent and treat pressure sores. In nursing homes the type of cushion on which the individual sits during the day should be written in the care plan.

Cushions

Cushions can be made of a variety of materials including silicore, foam, gel, fluid and air (Fig. 10.8). Depending on the material used and their construction, cushions will be suitable for different levels of risk. In nursing homes the registered nurse will ensure that the cushions provided are suitable for the individual patients. In residential homes carers can seek advice from district nursing staff.

Silicore cushions are padded cushions covered in fabric. They

Fig. 10.8   Range of cushions. (Courtesy Huntleigh Healthcare.)

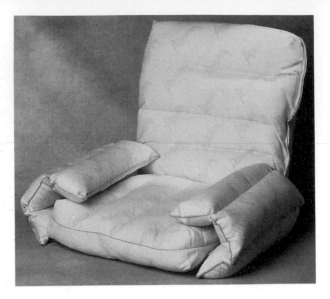

Fig. 10.9 Silicore cushion and Silicore wheelchair cushion. (Courtesy Huntleigh Healthcare.)

are used for comfort only. They can be machine washed and dried. Some have a waterproof side or seat which can be wiped clean. Special silicore cushions are designed to fit into wheelchairs (Fig. 10.9).

Foam cushions come in varying densities and can be made of different kinds of foam. They are light and simple to use. Some

Fig. 10.10 Fluid cushion. (Courtesy Huntleigh Healthcare.)

Fig. 10.11   Alternating air cushion. (Courtesy Huntleigh Healthcare.)

have a moulded surface which helps the cushion conform better to body shape and reduces shear. Some have a special core which allows air to circulate and prevents heat building up.

Gel cushions may be solid or fluid and are sometimes combined with foam to make them lighter. Fluid cushions (Fig. 10.10) can also be filled with foam in a way that has a dampening effect on the flow of fluid or to provide support for a fluid filled pad.

Alternating air cushions (Fig. 10.11) are designed to relieve pressure from the seating surface. Like pressure relieving mattresses their cells inflate and deflate in sequence to either support or relieve pressure from this area. They are either mains operated or powered by battery packs.

Heel protectors
Heel protectors (Fig. 10.12) are aids used to protect the heels of

Fig. 10.12   Heel protectors. (Courtesy Huntleigh Healthcare.)

patients who are very frail and at high risk of developing pressure
sores. They are made of either sheepskin (real or synthetic) or
silicore fibre, and are held in place with Velcro straps. They help
reduce and relieve pressure.

Heel blocks are made of soft foam and have a U shape in the
middle. The ankle fits into the U shape and the heels are held up
and do not touch the mattress. Heel blocks can only be used when
the patient is sitting up or lying on his back. Heel protectors are
used when the patient is lying on his side.

Elbow protectors

Elbow protectors (Fig. 10.13) are designed to protect elbows.
They are also made of sheepskin or silicore and are held in place
with Velcro straps.

Fig. 10.13   Elbow protectors. (Courtesy Huntleigh Healthcare.)

Treating pressure sores

Carers who fear that a patient is developing a pressure sore should
always seek professional help and advice from a nurse or doctor.
In most cases nurses will be responsible for treating the pressure
sore. The nurse will assess the sore and a plan of treatment will be
drawn up. This will involve changing the patient's position regularly; special mattresses, cushions and pressure relieving aids
may be used. The pressure sore will be covered with a protective
dressing to keep the wound clean and prevent it from drying out.
Wounds of all types, including pressure sores, are now known to
heal more quickly if they are kept warm and moist. Carers will be
involved in helping carry out the plan of care.

Caring for the whole person

People develop pressure sores because they are unable to move and relieve pressure. Illness can make a person more at risk of developing a pressure sore and the patient's doctor will treat any illness which could contribute to the development of a pressure sore.

If pressure sores are to be prevented it is important that the individual eats a healthy diet and has sufficient food and vitamins to prevent the skin breaking down. Older people who feel unwell may be reluctant to eat. The carer has an important role to play in informing trained staff if an individual has gone off their food. Carers can also find out what food the older person is fond of and inform other members of staff about their likes and dislikes.

It is important that the individual drinks enough fluid. The carer can encourage the older person to drink and can ensure that they have drinks that they like. Other members of staff should be informed about the individual's likes and dislikes. Further details on diet and fluids are given in Chapter 12.

Summary

Older people are more at risk of developing pressure sores than younger people. People living in homes are more at risk than those who live in their own homes. Pressure sores can be uncomfortable and painful for some patients; for others they can be life threatening. Most pressure sores can be prevented.

Some people living in homes are more frail than others. Assessment enables nurses to work out the individual's degree of risk of developing pressure sores, and to develop a plan of care. This enables the nurse to decide which type of mattresses, cushions and aids are required. The nurse should discuss the plan of care with the individual and obtain their consent and co-operation. Carers should be aware of the plan of care and should work with qualified staff in nursing homes, and under the direction of district nurses in residential homes, to prevent individuals developing pressure sores.

Portfolio preparation

- Check how many patients in your home are at risk of developing pressure sores because of immobility, incontinence or other risk factors.

- Find out which scale trained staff use to identify patients at risk. If you work in a residential home and do not use a scale, ask the district nurses which scale they use for assessing patients in the home whom they treat.
- Find out what aids are available within the home to prevent pressure sores, and list these.
- Ask if you can copy a care plan giving details of methods used to prevent pressure sores developing. Remember to remove the person's name from your copy to preserve confidentiality.

Further information

A number of wound care companies produce leaflets and information which carers may find of interest. Details of some of these are given below.

Convatec
Harrington House
Milton Road
Ickenham
Uxbridge UB10 8PU.
Help-line 0800 289738.

Convatec produce a useful booklet, *Pressure Sore Blueprint.* This is available free of charge. They also run a wound care help-line.

A range of educational material is available from:

Coloplast
Peterborough Business Park
Peterborough
Cambs. PE2 6FX.
Telephone 01733 392000.

Johnson & Johnson Medical
Coronation Road
Ascot
Berkshire SL5 9EY.
Telephone 01344 871000.

Pharma-plast Limited
Steriseal Division
Thornhill Road
Redditch
Worcester B98 9NL.
Telephone 01527 64222.

Smith & Nephew Healthcare
S&N Healthcare House
Goulton
Hull
HU3 4DJ.
Telephone 01482 222200.

Huntleigh Healthcare
310–312 Dallow Road
Luton
Bedfordshire LU1 1TD
Telephone 01582 413104

Reference

(1)   Registered Homes Act 1984 (1988). HMSO London.

Chapter 11

Personal Care and Hygiene

Introduction

This chapter deals with personal care. It includes:

- bathing
- making bathing a pleasure
- persuading the reluctant patient to bathe
- using hoists
- safety and privacy in the bathroom
- showers, assisted washes and bedbaths
- skin care, including skin care for incontinent patients and the use of barrier creams
- mouth care including care of dentures and natural teeth
- nail care including chiropody treatment
- hair care and hairdressing
- shaving
- choosing clothing and dressing
- cosmetics

Looking good and feeling good

People of all ages like to feel and look good. Many older people who have been in hospital arrive in homes wearing nightclothes and looking ill and tired. When the person is dressed in her normal clothes, has her hair set and is wearing make-up, she feels and looks much better. When we feel dirty, untidy and under the weather, bathing and making the effort to look good make us feel so much better.

Many older people who have just undergone surgery, for example for a fractured femur, feel worn out and fed up. Often they are unable to wash, dress and care for themselves without help. The carer, by helping the older person to bathe, care for her hair and nails and to dress, can make a real difference to the individual's morale. Suddenly the experience of coming into a home is not as bad as the individual feared. She is being helped to care for herself and is beginning to feel human once more. It has been said that the role of the nurse is to do for the patient what they would do for themselves if they had the strength and the will. Helping people to care for their personal appearance is not about helping patients to look or appear as we would wish, but as they would wish.

Bathing

Nowadays most of us take for granted our bathrooms with a supply of constant hot water. Many older people, though, grew up without such luxuries. They grew up in homes without bathrooms, central heating or hot water. People who did not have bathrooms either heated up water and bathed in a tin bath in front of a fire in the living room, or they visited the public baths. This involved much more effort than going upstairs and running a bath and so many older people bathed much less frequently than we do now.

How often a person baths is a personal choice. Some older people prefer to bath each day, whilst others feel that bathing twice a week is adequate. Bathing every day can help some patients to feel fresh and clear, for example those who perspire heavily or who suffer from incontinence. No harm, however, will come to most people if they do not bath every day. The decision of how often to bath should be the older person's, and whilst a carer can persuade an older person to bath, no older person should be bullied into bathing if they do not wish to do so. Bathing should be a pleasure and not a hurried chore. Carers who take the time and trouble to make the patient's bath a pleasant experience will find that the older person will look forward to the next bath.

Making bathing a pleasure

Many older people living in homes require help to bath. Even people who can bath without help depend on carers to ensure that the bathroom is safe, warm and comfortable. In many homes bathrooms become used as storerooms and fill up with boxes, broken chairs, commodes and other equipment. Carers should make sure that the bathroom is not used as a store room. Imagine how you would feel bathing in a room full of junk. Ask senior staff if equipment can be stored elsewhere. Keeping the bathroom clear makes it less likely that older people or carers using the bathroom will have an accident.

Often the bathroom window is left open and the room becomes cold. Carers should check that the window is closed before running the bath. The bathroom radiator should be turned on; carers who find the bathroom hot should remember that the patient who has bathed will find it much cooler.

The bath water should be the correct temperature. The carer should ask the individual how they like the water. Carers should always check the water temperature with an elbow before helping a patient into the bath. In some homes carers use bath thermometers. This avoids the risk of scalding. Patients who are confused may be unable to tell carers if the water is too hot. Patients who have no feeling in part of their body may not feel water that is too hot. In 1994 33 older people in hospital, nursing and residential homes suffered from serious burns because the water they were bathing in was too hot.

The water should be deep enough to wash in. Some staff attempt to bath patients in a few inches of water.

Bubble baths and bath oils

Many people like to use scented bubble bath or bath oils in the bath. Bubble bath adds a touch of luxury and many people enjoy using it. Some bubble baths, though, can make an older person's skin very dry; moisturising cream bubble bath can prevent this. Some older people have very sensitive skin and bubble bath can make it itch. It is now possible to buy bubble baths especially for people with sensitive skin. These avoid using agents such as lanolin, which can cause allergies. Most supermarkets sell their own brand of sensitive skin bubble bath and many other companies make them too. Carers can either ask relatives to buy these, can buy them for the older person who can pay from their personal allowance, or can take the older person shopping. This will depend on the policy of the home. Some older people continue to suffer from dry or sensitive skin despite these measures and carers should seek professional advice. The patient's doctor may prescribe special bubble bath designed for patients with very sensitive skin.

Bath oils should be used with caution. Some make the skin very slippery. This does not normally cause a problem if the older person is helped in and out of the bath by using a hoist. If the individual only requires a hand to step out of the bath then bath oils which can make the skin, the bath and even a bath mat slippery, should be used with care.

Soap

Some older people prefer to wash with soap instead of using bubble bath, shower gel and foam washes. Most people can use soap without any ill effects. Some older people who have dry skin find that soap makes it even drier. It is now possible to buy soaps which have moisturising cream in them; using these prevents the skin becoming dry. People with sensitive skin can use unperfumed soaps made specially for sensitive skins. If these do not help, the patient's doctor can prescribe special soap.

Talcum powder

Many older people like to use talcum powder after drying their skin. Some older people may find that heavily perfumed talc makes their skin itch. Using either baby powder or unscented talcum powder can prevent this problem.

Persuading the reluctant patient to bath

Some older people may be reluctant to bath. They may have found that the bath was rushed and was an ordeal rather than a pleasure. Male patients may be embarrassed to appear naked in front of a young female carer. Some older people need help to get in and out of the bath but may not like to ask as they do not want to 'appear a nuisance' or 'trouble the staff'. Some older people may be suffering from pain and may fear that getting in and out of the bath will make it worse. Others may feel that there is no opportunity to bathe in private. Carers should take the time and trouble to find out why the older person is reluctant and should try to make bathing as pleasant an experience as possible. If the older person likes a long leisurely soak but the bathrooms are busy in the morning, perhaps the carer could suggest a bath in the afternoon or evening when the home is not so busy. If the individual does not wish to bath carers should respect the person's wishes.

Using hoists – legal requirements

Hoists are often used to help older people get in and out of the bath safely. Many older people living in nursing and residential homes are unable to get in and out of the bath without assistance. People who are mobile and merely require a steadying hand to get in and out of the bath do not require hoists. Other older people are unable to stand, bend or get into the bath unless they are lifted.

In the past, staff in some homes were expected to lift older people in and out of the bath without hoists. Sometimes, if an individual was very disabled or heavy, two people had to lift the individual out. Many bathrooms in homes are small and carers often had difficulty in lifting because there was not enough room. Carers were in danger of injuring their backs and at risk of injuring the patient.

In January 1993 six European Community directives were introduced to improve health and safety. The Manual Handling

Loads Directive states that: 'The employer shall have a duty to ensure the safety and health of all workers in every aspect of work'. Under UK[1] and European law, employers have a duty to introduce policies to assess the risk of injury if staff lift people or objects. Homes should have policies which assess how heavy patients are and whether they can bear any of their own weight. Each patient who requires lifting must have an assessment carried out. A plan of care must be drawn up which instructs staff how to lift the individual and what equipment should be used.

Patients who are unable to bear any of their own weight must not be lifted unless hoists are used. Employers who expect staff to lift patients in and out of the bath and do not provide hoists are acting illegally.

Two different types of hoist are normally used to bath patients.

Fig. 11.1 Hoist with wheels.

The first is a mobile hoist, which is normally on wheels and is wheeled to the patient's bed (Fig. 11.1). The patient is transferred onto the hoist and wheeled to the bathroom. The hoist is attached to an upright column which is screwed to the floor and the hoist is raised off the ground by turning a handle. The section of the hoist which has the wheels is detached, and the chair section is placed over the bath (Fig. 11.2). The patient is lowered into the bath.

Fig. 11.2   Hoist ready to be lowered into bath.

The second type is a fixed hoist, which is a chair with a lifting column and a base plate screwed to the floor (Fig. 11.3). This type is more suitable for patients who are not severely disabled. The patient walks or is wheeled into the bathroom, and is then helped to transfer into the hoist. The hoist is raised and positioned over the bath, and the patient is lowered into the bath.

Fixed hoists are more suitable for more able patients. The disadvantage of fixed hoists is that an individual who requires help to transfer must be transferred from chair to wheelchair to hoist and then back again. Using a mobile hoist reduces the number of transfers required. Mobile hoists, though, can cost three times as much as fixed hoists. They also take up more room. In homes which have not been purpose built, bathrooms are often small and there may not be enough room for a mobile hoist.

Fig. 11.3   Fixed hoist.

Few residential homes will have mobile hoists because patients are less disabled than those in nursing homes. Nursing homes should have facilities for bathing very disabled patients. A mobile hoist or a special type of bath such as a Parker bath (Fig. 11.4) should be provided. Using special equipment such as hoists and Parker baths protects both patients and staff from injury. Carers

Fig. 11.4   Parker bath.

should check which type of hoists are available in their workplace and should make sure they know how to operate them. Details of equipment required to lift the individual who cannot bear part of his or her weight should be written on the care plan .

Further information on lifting and handling is given in Chapter 9.

Safety and privacy in the bathroom

Most people take it for granted that they can enjoy a bath in peace without interruptions. Most people lock the bathroom door and enjoy a relaxing bath. How many patients in homes can enjoy peace and privacy whilst bathing? In some homes staff leave the bathroom door ajar so that they can 'keep an eye on' the older person. In other homes staff have strict instructions that patients must not be left alone in the bathroom, 'in the interests of safety'. Yet the nursing or residential home is the patient's home and all over the country older people bath without being watched.

Some patients, though, are very frail and it would not be safe to leave them alone. Some individuals who suffer from dementia and are confused could try to get up and fall, or could slip over and drown. In 1994 there were 17 cases of older people who suffered injury whilst bathing in hospitals and homes.

How can staff respect the patient's privacy and dignity and yet prevent accidents? It is important to realise that very few older people are at risk of injuring themselves whilst bathing. Staff have a duty of care and any member of staff who left a patient unattended in the bath *knowing that the patient was at risk of injury* would have failed in that duty of care. Older people living in homes have differing abilities. An older person who lives in a home and who requires assistance to get in and out of the bath has the same right to privacy as a person living in their own home. If the older person can be safely left in the bath then carers should respect the individual's right to privacy. However, if the older person is confused and might turn on the hot tap and scald herself, the carer would be failing to provide proper care if she failed to remain with the patient. If the older person suffers from a disease which may cause her to faint or lose consciousness, the carer should remain with the patient to ensure that she is safe.

In nursing homes the care plan should include details of how much assistance the individual requires and what measures are required to maintain safety. In residential and nursing homes, if carers are not sure whether it is safe to leave a patient they should ask senior staff. The charity Counsel and Care has produced a book about balancing patient safety and providing dignity and privacy[2].

Showers

Many new homes have shower rooms which have been specially designed for patients. Unfortunately many shower rooms are not used as many older people are reluctant to use showers because they have not used them before. Many staff who have worked in older homes without showers prefer not to use showers.

But showers can be refreshing and modern specially designed showers enable older people to wash themselves. Some showers are in specially designed rooms with slightly sloping floors. Special shower seats are provided so that the individual can shower sitting down. Often shower controls have been placed at sitting height and the showers have thermostatic valves to prevent scalding.

Shower chairs with wheels are available so that patients who cannot walk can be wheeled into the shower room where they can shower independently if possible, or carers can shower them if necessary.

Some showers are not purpose built and resemble ordinary shower cubicles. Placing a plastic chair in the cubicle, such as the type of stacking chair homes often provide for visits, can allow older people who are unable to stand to use the shower. Showers should have non-slip flooring, but even some of this can become quite slippery when wet. Carers should help older people who are in danger of slipping, when they are going in and out of the shower. If the shower does not have a thermostatic valve which prevents the risk of scalding, carers should adjust the water temperature and remain with the patient to check that the water does not get too hot.

Soap can be difficult to keep hold of in the shower, especially for older people who may have suffered from strokes or who have arthritic hands. Soap on a rope can be hooked around the shower control (if at sitting height) or on a hook, to make washing easier. Some patients prefer to use shower gels or body washes which can also be used as shampoos. These are available in sensitive skin and non-perfumed versions for people who have dry and sensitive skin.

Assisted washes

Individuals who do not wish to bath or shower each day may need help to wash. They may need help to get soap, flannels, talc, deodorant and clothing ready. If everything is ready before the wash, the water will not get cold. The carer can help the person to the wash basin and help them to wash. It is safer for most older people to wash sitting in a chair.

The wash basin may be too high to allow the person to use it comfortably when seated. In this case the carer can bring a bowl of warm water. The person remains seated in the chair and the water is placed on a bed table. It is important to make sure that the person is able to wash in private. If the person shares a room with another person, curtains should be drawn around the patient. If the room is overlooked, the window curtains should be drawn. If the person has a single room it may have a 'Do not disturb' or 'Engaged' sign on the outside; this should be used so that visitors do not enter and embarrass the person who is washing.

The individual may require help to undress. Carers should encourage the older person to wash as much of the body as they can manage. Often older people who require assisted washes find it difficult to wash the back, bottom, lower legs and feet. The carer can wash these areas, dry them thoroughly, apply powder if the patient uses it and help put on any clothing which the individual is unable to manage.

Bed baths

Patients who are very frail and ill may require a bed bath. This is simply a name for a wash which is carried out in bed. It may be carried out by one or two members of staff depending on the home's policies, staffing levels and how much care the patient requires.

Towels, flannels, soap, talcum powder, deodorant and any other toiletries are removed from the patient's locker, with the patient's permission, and placed on the bed table. A bowl of water is brought to the bedside. The bed curtains are drawn, the room door closed and window curtains drawn if the room is overlooked. The carer explains that she is going to wash the patient and make her more comfortable.

The bedclothes or duvet are removed and the patient is covered with a sheet, blanket or large towel depending on the home's policy and the temperature. If it is a hot sticky summer's day, a blanket could be hot and uncomfortable. On a chilly winter's morning, a sheet would not be warm enough.

Two flannels are used for washing. One, usually a light colour, is used for the face. Another, usually a darker colour, is used for the body. Many people, especially women, do not use soap on their faces and only wash the face with plain water. The carer should ask the patient if she normally washes her face with soap.

The carer then folds the cover back and washes the neck, arms, chest and abdomen. The flannel is soaped and an area of the body washed. The flannel is then rinsed and the area of the body rinsed and dried. Talcum powder is applied if the person wishes. It is easy to use too much talcum powder if using it directly from the container. This can be uncomfortable and can cause skin irritation. If too much talcum powder is used in skin folds, such as under the arms or under the breasts, the powder can cake. Placing talcum powder on a powder puff and then applying it to the skin prevents this, as it is easier to avoid putting too much on. Supermarkets and chemists sell powder puffs designed for applying talc.

If the patient can sit forward, the carer can ask her to do so and wash her back. Patients who are able to do so should be encouraged to wash their own genital area. If the patient is unable to assist the carer by sitting up, a second member of staff can help the carer to lie the patient down and roll her over onto her side. Staff should explain what they are going to do and obtain the patient's consent before moving her. The front of the patient's body is covered and the back, buttocks and the area between the legs (perineum) is washed and dried. The patient may like to have powder on her back.

It is not advisable to put powder on the perineal area or the groin as the powder can cake. This is a particular problem with incontinent patients. If the patient is incontinent a barrier cream may be applied *lightly* to the buttocks and perineum. Too much cream interferes with the action of incontinence pads. Further details on caring for the skin of incontinent patients is given later in this chapter.

The water should then be changed. This is important because the water will have become cooler and full of soap suds. The back of the legs are then washed and the patient is rolled over onto her back. The top half of the patient's body is covered and the remaining parts of the lower front of the body washed, dried and powder applied if the patient wishes.

Some staff prefer to turn the patient onto her back before changing the water. This practice will vary depending on the patient's condition. A person with breathing difficulties will find it easier to breathe if sat up whilst other patients may be safer left on their sides. Some staff prefer to lift and wash the front of the leg and then lift it to wash the back. This again will depend on the person's condition as this can be uncomfortable for arthritic patients. Although techniques vary, the basic principles remain the same. It is important to ensure that the person's body remains covered and that only the part being washed is exposed.

The patient is then dressed or helped to dress in clean night-clothes.

If the patient is well enough she can be helped to sit in a chair while bed linen is changed and the bed made. The carer can then help the patient to clean teeth or dentures, to comb and style hair, and to apply make-up if she wishes. Male patients may require help with shaving.

In some homes carers may find that the bed bathing technique varies. Some staff use two bowls of water to carry out a bed bath, one for washing and the other for rinsing. Both bowls of water will still require changing as the water will become cooler.

It is important that carers remember that although bed bathing techniques differ, the aims remain the same. The patient's dignity and privacy should be protected at all times. The patient should be covered to prevent her from becoming cold. The patient's own preferences should be sought. One important part of bed bathing is sometimes forgotten – the patient. Bed bathing a patient gives the carer an important opportunity to get to know the patient and to communicate with her. Often patients confide their worries and fears during a bed bath. A patient may tell the carer that her arthritis seems to be getting worse and that the pain killers do not seem to be doing so much good these days. Another might confide that the new tablets make her feel sick. It is important that carers share such information with professional staff. The doctor may be able to change the pain killers or increase the dose so that the patient is no longer in pain. The patient whose tablets are making her feel sick may be able to have a different type of tablets.

Skin care

Skin is a waterproof protective covering. It is sensitive to heat, cold, touch and pressure. Skin is elastic and stretches, and it grows and contracts as a person becomes fatter or thinner. Healthy skin protects the body against infection. As people age, their skin becomes less elastic and tends to wrinkle. The skin becomes drier and thinner and can be more easily damaged than the skin of younger people. Certain medicines, such as steroids and anti-inflammatory drugs given to treat arthritis, affect the skin. These medicines can cause the skin to be very easily damaged.

When the skin is damaged it is no longer able to prevent infection. Dry skin can become damaged more easily than healthy skin. Many older people suffer from very dry skin, and it is usually worst on the legs and arms. Older people's skin is often more sensitive than younger people's. Carers should advise older people with sensitive and dry skin to avoid using heavily perfumed soaps and bubble baths. Special bubble baths, soaps and talcum can now be bought in most supermarkets and chemists.

Caring for dry skin

People who have dry skin may have found their own solutions. Some patients have their own favourite moisturisers which they have been using for years. Sometimes the older person is no longer able to bend down and apply moisturiser to the legs or another part of the body. Carers should offer to do this if the older person can no longer manage.

Sometimes the skin is so dry that normal moisturisers and oils are not effective. In this case carers should seek professional advice. The patient's doctor may prescribe special moisturising creams. These should normally be applied after a bath. Some creams are more effective if applied to damp skin. Trained nurses will be able to offer advice and show carers how to apply these moisturising creams. Patients who require specially prescribed creams should have this noted in their care plan in nursing homes. A record should also be kept in residential homes. The carer who is applying these creams will soon see if the prescribed cream is effective. She should inform professional staff and colleagues about the condition of the patient's skin. If the skin is not improving the patient's doctor will visit again and may prescribe a different cream. In very severe cases the patient's doctor may ask a skin specialist or dermatologist to see the patient.

Caring for the skin of incontinent patients

Patients who suffer from incontinence can easily develop inflamed skin (dermatitis) because the skin is in contact with urine. Patients who are incontinent of faeces as well as urine are at high risk of developing sore inflamed skin. This inflamed skin can become infected and can make patients more at risk of developing pressure sores. Patients who are incontinent should be washed each time they have been incontinent. Washing removes traces of urine from the skin. Urine can irritate the skin and cause soreness.

Many incontinent patients have their genital area and bottom washed six or seven times each day. If the carer uses soap each time, the patient's skin can soon become very dry. Dry skin can develop small cracks and can easily become infected. It is recommended that carers wash the skin using soap and water only two or three times each day. The soap used should be mild and unperfumed. At other times the patient's skin should be cleaned with plain water.

Barrier creams – are they necessary?

Barrier creams are creams which are used to coat the skin and provide a protective barrier which prevents the skin becoming soggy and sore. Some nurses who specialise in the care of patients with continence problems (continence advisers) state that barrier creams should only be used if the patient's skin is becoming sore. Others state that prevention is better than cure. Many trained nurses disagree on when barrier creams should be used.

Any patient who is incontinent of faeces and urine should have a barrier cream applied at all times. This will help prevent the skin becoming sore when faeces and urine mix to form ammonia, which can cause skin damage very quickly. Any patient who has red, inflamed skin should have a barrier cream applied. In the home where I work barrier cream is routinely applied to the bottom and genital area of all patients who suffer from incontinence. Skin problems are rare.

Which barrier cream is best?

There are more than 50 different barrier creams available. Some continence advisers recommend using petroleum jelly. This forms a waterproof barrier and stops urine sticking to the skin. Others recommend zinc and castor oil cream and others will recommend different preparations. People are individuals and a cream that is effective and protects one person's skin may not be so effective on another person's skin. Many homes use a few different products. These are prescribed by the doctor for the individual. Each patient who requires a barrier cream should have their own labelled cream, which should be used only for that person. Sharing or borrowing creams increases the risk of infection. If an individual's skin is becoming sore or is failing to improve despite a cream being used, carers should seek professional advice. The individual may have developed a skin infection (cellulitis), and prompt treatment can prevent further complications from developing.

Mouth care

Mouth care is an area of caring that is often forgotten, carried out poorly or thought to be of little importance. Mouth care, though, is very important. The patient who has a toothache, sore gums because dentures are rubbing or a sore tongue because a broken tooth is catching on it, may not wish to eat or drink. Without sufficient food and fluids the patient will become weaker and less able to fight off illness. A sore mouth can make a person feel miserable and depressed. It has been said that the best way of judging the quality of care is to check the mouths of patients.

Caring for natural teeth

Many older people living in homes no longer have any natural teeth. Some older people, though, have some or all of their own teeth. Patients admitted to nursing homes will have a nursing history taken before they are admitted. This will have information about the patient's teeth, dentures or partial dentures written on it. In residential homes carers will have to enquire.

Older people who have their own teeth should care for them normally. The teeth should be brushed morning and evening; some forgetful patients may need reminding. Some patients who are unable to walk to the wash basin will require a tooth mug with water, a dish to rinse their mouths into, and their toothbrush and toothpaste. Some older people are unable to brush their teeth and carers may have to do it for them. Try practising by brushing a colleague's teeth. You can then swap roles and discuss it when you have finished.

People who have their natural teeth should continue to have six-monthly dental check-ups and may require dental treatment such as fillings and crowns. Dental check-ups can be carried out either at the dental surgery or at the home. Dentists who provide dental care to the home may be either dentists who practice locally or part of the community dental service. Find out what the dental arrangements are in your home.

As people age, their teeth are more at risk of breaking or cracking. People who have their own teeth should be advised not to eat hard sweets such as boiled sweets and sugared almonds, as crunching on these can cause teeth to break.

Caring for dentures

Caring for dentures is as important as caring for natural teeth. People who are unable to clean their dentures can have food debris building up under them. This can cause gums to become sore and inflamed. Dentures should be cleaned morning and evening with a toothbrush and toothpaste. Some older people do not remove dentures but clean them while they are in the mouth. It is not possible to clean the inner part of the dentures or the top palate without removing them. Individuals should be advised to remove dentures so that they can be cleaned properly.

Many older people prefer to remove dentures and soak them overnight. Dentures can be soaked in either plain water or denture cleaning tablets. The denture pot is filled with warm water and the denture cleaning tablet is added. *Cleaned* dentures are soaked overnight. Denture cleaning tablets contain a mild bleach and this removes stains such as coffee and tea. It can be difficult to remove such stains by brushing. If an older person who wears dentures complains of sore gums, professional advice should be sought. The denture may have become ill fitting and is rubbing. The dentist can treat this and adjust, alter, or make new dentures if required.

Mouth care for the frail patient

Patients who are very ill or frail may depend on staff to clean their mouths. Many older people who are unwell are unable to tolerate their dentures. The person who feels sick may find having the dentures out is more comfortable. Other patients prefer to continue to wear their dentures. Denture care is as given above.

The frail patient should be offered mouthwashes. There are many different types available. Dentists now recommend that plain water is offered as a mouthwash. Mouthwashes, research has discovered, can kill off bacteria in the mouth which keep the mouth healthy. Using mouthwashes can cause sore mouths and some patients can develop oral thrush if they are used. Normally, unless a mouthwash has been especially prescribed by the person's doctor, the mouth is only rinsed with plain water.

Some patients are so ill that they are unable to rinse their mouths with water. Some homes have mouth care trays, which have special swabs to clean out the mouth. These are sticks with a piece of pink foam on top. The foam is dipped into water and then inserted into the patient's mouth. Some homes no longer use these. There have been cases where the foam has come off the stick or has been bitten off by the patient. The foam has been inhaled in a few cases and emergency hospital treatment required to remove the foam from the lung. In some homes pre-moistened swabs are available. There have been no reports of problems with their use.

The aim of mouth care in very frail patients is to remove food debris and traces of milky fluids from the mouth. Dentists now recommend that gauze moistened in water is wrapped around a gloved finger, and used to gently clean the mouth. The inside of the mouth can be wiped with glycerine after cleaning. This keeps the mouth moist and prevents soreness. Lips can become dry, sore and cracked when people are very ill. Petroleum jelly or lip salve prevents this and keeps the individual feeling comfortable.

Nail care

Many older people have difficulty in caring for their nails. People who suffer from arthritis can find it difficult to use scissors or nail clippers because their hands can no longer manage fine movements. People with poor eyesight cannot see well enough to cut or file nails. People suffering from Parkinson's disease often suffer from fine tremors which make nail care difficult. People who have suffered from strokes and can only use one hand find it impossible to care for their nails. One survey of fit and healthy people over the age of 85 found that few people of this age could manage to bend down and cut their own toe nails.

Uncared for finger nails can become dirty and torn and people with nails like this look uncared for and dishevelled. Many people prefer to have their nails cut with nail scissors or clippers and kept short. Some women though prefer to keep their nails longer and have them filed, manicured and painted with nail varnish. Carers should ask individuals how they prefer to have their finger nails and should not assume that all older women like short nails.

Grace Adams felt depressed when she had to give up her home and enter a nursing home. Her carer noticed that her nails were long and dirty and offered to attend to them. Grace explained that she had always been proud of her hands and nails and had kept her nails long, manicured and painted red all of her adult life. Having attractive hands and nails made her feel feminine and attractive. One of the things that had upset her most was that she was unable to care for her hands and paint her nails after her stroke. Her carer, June, soaked her hands in a bowl of water, scrubbed the dirt from beneath her nails, and pushed back the ragged cuticles surrounding the nails with a 'Cutipen'. She then applied hand cream to the hands and painted Grace's nails with two coats of nail varnish and applied a top coat of varnish. Grace felt like an attractive woman again and not a 'dishevelled old dear with dirty nails'. Caring for the patient's nails can have an important effect on morale. The carer gets a great feeling of satisfaction from making a patient feel better.

Many older people are unable to cut their own toe nails and many are admitted to homes with nails that have become so long they are curling over and cutting into the toes. Some older people have toe nails which are very thick and difficult to cut. Toe nails become thicker when circulation to the feet is poor. It is almost impossible to cut thickened toe nails with ordinary nail scissors. Older people who do not have thickened toe nails can have their toe nails cut with ordinary nail scissors. Carers should check what the policy is for cutting the nails of people who have thickened toe nails. In some nursing homes these nails are cut by qualified staff. The home should have strong nail scissors, clippers and files so that these nails can be cut. In other homes qualified nurses do not cut nails but arrange for the chiropodist to call and do it.

Chiropodists

Many chiropodists work with foot care assistants and will often arrange for a foot care assistant to come to the home and cut nails. Chiropodists will call and treat patients who have foot problems such as ingrowing toe nails, corns and bunions. The chiropodist who visits the home may be either a private chiropodist or one employed by the local NHS community trust. Private chiropodists charge either by the session (usually three quarters of an hour) or charge for each patient seen. If your home uses a private chiropodist find out how much each treatment costs. In most homes patients pay these charges as they are seldom included in home fees except in the most expensive of private homes. There is no charge for NHS chiropody but some areas do not have enough chiropody staff and it can be difficult to arrange regular visits.

Hair care

As people age, the hair loses the pigment which gives us our hair colour. Hair becomes grey or white. White hair is coarser in texture and drier. Hair thins with age. Men may lose all their hair and become bald. The scalp becomes drier and more sensitive with age. Older people very rarely have greasy hair and usually a shampoo once or twice each week will keep the hair clean. Washing the hair daily will make dry hair and a dry scalp even drier. Older people should be encouraged or helped to wash their hair once or twice a week. If the hair is dry, a mild shampoo for dry hair should be used. Many female patients have their hair permed regularly. Perming makes the hair dry. Patients who have perms should use a conditioner after shampooing, to prevent the hair becoming dry and brittle and make it easier to comb and style. Some patients prefer to use a shampoo and conditioner in one. If this is used then one specially for dry hair should be chosen.

If a patient is unwell and unable to have a shampoo, a dry shampoo can be used to freshen up the hair. Dry shampoos can be purchased in chemists and are powders which are puffed onto the hair through an applicator and then brushed out. They remove dirt and debris from the hair but do not tire a person out when she is feeling unwell. Dry shampoos are not intended to be used long term. They can be useful if someone is feeling under the weather, perhaps because of a chest infection or an illness.

Some older people develop dry, flaking and itching scalps; in extreme cases sores can form on the scalp and these can bleed. If an individual develops a dry, flaking, itchy scalp, professional advice should be sought. The patient's doctor will normally prescribe a shampoo containing coal tar (to prevent the flaking and treat the itching) and coconut oil (to treat the dryness). The patient's hair is normally shampooed daily and the shampoo left on for 10–15 minutes; as the condition improves the hair is washed less frequently, until it is washed once or twice each week. Perming lotions, tints and setting lotions should not be used until the patient's doctor has agreed that the scalp is normal. The hairdresser should be informed about any problems with a patient's scalp and will test each lotion on the individual's forearm to make sure that the person is not allergic to it, before using it on the person's hair.

Hairdressing

For many women a trip to the hairdressers is a treat. Women feel good when their hair looks good. Having a hairdo is important to many older women. Most homes have a hairdresser who visits once or twice a week and washes, cuts, perms, shampoos and sets hair for female patients. Male patients have their hair cut.

It is important that carers realise that women do not stop caring about their appearance as they age. Carers can help patients keep their hair looking nice between styles. Some people have fine hair

Fig. 11.5 Patient having her hair dressed.

and find that wearing a hair net helps keep a set looking good for longer. The carer can help the individual put on her hair net before going to sleep if she can no longer manage this. When the carer is helping the individual to wash and dress she should remember to help comb and style hair if the person has difficulty.

Shaving

Men, especially older men, often feel dirty and scruffy if they are unshaven. Many male patients have difficulty shaving themselves. A stroke can cause an older person to lose the use of one hand. Parkinson's disease can cause tremor. Poor eyesight can make it difficult to see well enough to shave.

Wet shaves

Many older men prefer to use a shaving stick and brush to make shaving foam. This is applied to the bristles to soften the hair. Shaving foam may contain perfume and people with sensitive skin can react to this and suffer from red and itchy skin. It is now possible to buy shaving sticks, foam and gel for sensitive skin. A razor is then used to remove hair.

Using a foam and a razor gives a closer shave then using an electric razor, and many male patients prefer a wet shave. Many carers fear cutting the patient's skin and so encourage the patient (or his relatives) to buy an electric razor. Wet shaving is not difficult (half of the adult population do it daily) and the carer should not be put off by fears of cutting the patient. If a male patient prefers to have a wet shave, carers should respect the individual's wishes. Senior staff can help and advise you in learning how to shave a male patient.

Electric razors

Many male patients, including those who have a tremor or can only use one hand, find it possible to shave using an electric razor. Electric razors can help an older person retain his independence. Each male patient should have his own razor. Carers should not 'borrow' another patient's electric razor to use on a patient whose own shaver is broken. Electric razors can cause very small cuts on the skin. If two people share a razor there is a risk of both developing a skin infection.

After-shave

Many patients like to use after-shave, but it contains perfume, alcohol and colourings and these can inflame the skin of some patients. Special after-shave made for people with sensitive skin can be used if ordinary after-shave irritates the skin.

Clothing

Our clothes say a lot about us, about our personality and our mood. Older people enjoy wearing clothes which they have chosen themselves. Clothing should be comfortable, attractive and practical. Many older people living in homes enjoy choosing their own clothes, yet in many homes clothes are not chosen and bought by the individual but by family and friends, or by carers if the older person has no family.

Choosing clothing

Some homes arrange trips into shopping centres so that older people can choose their own clothes. The local St John Ambulance, Red Cross or Dial-A-Ride service often provide transport to enable people to make shopping trips. Some large stores have special open evenings for disabled people. Other large stores are willing to open for an extra hour and provide facilities for disabled and elderly people to shop after normal shopping hours. Some homes have companies come in with a selection of clothing and elderly people can select and try on clothes in the home. What arrangements has your home made to enable patients to choose their own clothing?

Advising disabled older people on choosing suitable clothing

Many disabled people have difficulty in dressing. Often choosing clothes which take account of the disability helps the older person to regain the ability to dress without help. Many women find:

- dresses which fasten at the front are easier to put on
- dresses and blouses with wide sleeves are easier to put on than those with tight sleeves
- skirts and trousers with elasticated waistbands are easier to put on and more comfortable to wear than those with buttons at the waistband
- A-line or full skirts are more comfortable to wear than straight skirts

People who have difficulty doing up buttons and fasteners may find that:

- large buttons are easier to fasten
- zips are easier to do up than fasteners
- elasticated trousers such as jogging pants may be more comfortable than other trousers
- Velcro can be used for fastenings on clothes

Helping people to help themselves

Many older people prefer to dress independently. Helping them to choose clothing which is easy to put on and fasten enables many older people to retain independence. Many people find that aids help them retain their independence, such as the 'Helping Hand', a metal tool which can help an older person to put on stockings unaided. If the carer feels that an older person might benefit from an aid she should consult senior staff who will take appropriate action.

Further reading

Jenkins J. (1992) *The clothes in question.* Scutari Press, Harrow. This book gives advice and information on choosing, adapting and caring for patients' clothes when they are living in homes.
Disabled Living Foundation (1994) *All dressed up.* Disabled Living Foundation, London. This book is full of practical advice and tips on choosing and adapting clothes. It also provides elderly people with advice on how to dress. There is a section on how to dress people who are unable to dress themselves.

Cosmetics

Some women living in nursing homes have been wearing cosmetics all their adult lives and feel naked without 'a touch of powder, rouge and lipstick'. Others prefer 'not to paint my face'. Carers should respect the individual's wishes. Some patients find it difficult to apply make-up because of failing eyesight. Using a magnifying mirror can make it easier for the person to see more clearly. Some patients may require help in putting on make-up, especially lipstick which can be difficult to apply if hands are not steady. People with sensitive skins can buy hypo-allergenic make-up which is less likely to cause allergies and skin reactions.

Summary

People of all ages enjoy looking and feeling good. Many older people living in homes require help with personal hygiene needs.

The aim of care is to help or meet the hygiene needs of the older person. The rewards are enormous. Older people who are helped to regain or maintain independence feel in control of their lives and are happier and more fulfilled. People who are helped to look and feel good are less likely to become depressed and ill. The carer has the satisfaction of doing her job to the best of her ability.

Portfolio preparation

- What facilities are available in your home to bath patients?
- Note ways in which you offer assistance whilst enabling the older person to maintain dignity and privacy.
- Find out how hairdressing services are organized within the home.
- Find out how dental services are arranged. Are patients seen routinely for six-monthly or annual check-ups or does the dentist only visit when problems arise?
- Find out how chiropody services are provided. Does the community chiropodist visit and provide footcare free of charge, or does a private chiropodist visit? If a private chiropodist visits, find out the cost of treatment and if this treatment is included in the home's fees.

References

(1)   Health and Safety Executive (1992) *Statutory Instrument no 2793, the manual handling operations guidance regulations*. HMSO, London.
(2)   Counsel & Care (1993) *The right to take risks*. Counsel & Care, London.

Chapter 12

Nutrition and Diet

Introduction

Food and fluids are more than just fuel for our bodies. Meal times can be relaxed pleasurable occasions. This chapter gives information on:

- the importance of fluids
- why some older people are at risk of becoming dehydrated
- normal fluid requirements
- helping and encouraging patients to drink
- recording fluid intake and output
- the importance of a healthy diet
- calories requirements
- what is a healthy diet
- vitamins and minerals
- special diets
- meeting the dietary needs of people from different cultures
- dietary supplements

The importance of fluids

Healthy people will die within three days if they do not have fluids. Fluid is essential to life. The human body is mostly water in healthy young adults. Women's bodies contain less fluid than men's because women carry more fat on their bodies and fat contains little fluid. The amount of fluid in the body lessens with age. The average older man's body is 55% fluid and the average older woman's body is 45% fluid.

Each day we lose fluid and if the fluid lost is not replaced the amount of fluid in the body is reduced. This process is known as dehydration. Each day the average person loses fluid in:

- urine – normally 1500 ml is produced
- breath – normally 400 ml of fluid is lost in the breath
- faeces – normally 100 ml of fluid is lost in faeces
- sweat – the amount of fluid lost in sweat will vary according to the temperature and how much the individual perspires.

It is important that the individual drinks enough fluid to replace fluids lost by the body. If the person does not drink sufficient fluids, the balance of chemicals (known as electrolytes) within the body is disturbed and this can lead to illness. People who do not drink enough are at risk of developing urine infections, are more likely to become constipated, have less resistance to infection and are at risk of developing infections, such as a chest infection, which can lead to serious ill health or even death.

Individuals who become dehydrated may become confused. Dehydration causes the blood to thicken and become more sticky (viscous). The blood is more likely to clot and blood clots can lead to strokes, heart attacks and blood clots in the legs (deep vein thrombosis). All of these can cause serious illness which can lead to the older person becoming more disabled. In some cases the older person may die as a result of the complications of dehydration.

Why older people living in homes may become dehydrated

Normally when it is hot or we are in danger of becoming dehydrated we become thirsty. Drinking restores the body's normal fluid balance. This is known as the thirst mechanism. As people age the thirst mechanism becomes less efficient and even when older people are becoming dehydrated they do not feel as thirsty as younger people. In hot weather or when we are in danger of becoming dehydrated, our kidneys respond by trying to conserve water. Less urine is produced. As people age the kidneys become less efficient at concentrating urine and conserving water.

Some people who live in nursing homes have problems communicating with carers. Even if they are thirsty they may have difficulty in asking staff for a drink. Some older people living in homes suffer from confusion and although they are thirsty they may have difficulty in understanding that this is the problem. Confusion gets worse if the individual does not have enough fluid. These patients depend on carers to leave a drink where they can reach it, perhaps on the patient's locker or table.

Some people are unable to manage to drink without help even if the drink is placed in front of them. People suffering from arthritis may be unable to hold or lift the cup. People with a tremor may drop the cup or glass. The person who has had a stroke or who has poor eyesight may be unable to see the glass.

Some people are reluctant to drink because they suffer from urinary incontinence and are afraid that they will have an accident if they drink. Some people have difficulty in swallowing because illness makes it difficult. People who have had strokes or have

Parkinson's disease or motor neurone disease may have difficulty in swallowing. The older person may not like the drink he has been given.

Some individuals may need more fluid than others. A person who has diabetes may pass much more urine than normal. The reasons for this are given later in the chapter.

The person may have a leg ulcer or pressure sore which can weep fluid and increase their fluid requirements.

The older person may be vomiting, or may have diarrhoea, or they may feel sick, perhaps because of the medication they are taking, or perhaps because of constipation.

How much fluid do older people normally require?

Older people normally require two litres of fluids each day. Check how much fluid a tea cup holds in your home. The average tea cup holds approximately 250 ml, but the cups in your home may be slightly larger or smaller than average. Remember when measuring how much a cup holds, that cups are not normally filled to the brim and most people do not drain their cups. Usually a little tea or coffee is left in the bottom of the cup. Check how much fluid the drinking glasses used in your home hold. The capacity of a drinking glass varies more than that of tea cups. Drinking glasses hold between 250 and 330 ml on average.

When do older people require extra fluids?

Most people require two litres of fluid each day but there are times when individuals require more fluid. If it is hot individuals will sweat more and will require extra fluid to prevent dehydration. When people have an infection the body fights it by raising the body temperature, because bacteria and viruses are usually killed by higher than normal body temperatures. When the body temperature rises the individual will sweat more and increased fluids are required to replace fluid lost in this way.

Normally approximately 100 ml of fluid is lost in faeces each day. If the older person has diarrhoea, the amount of fluid lost from the bowel increases. Extra fluid is needed to replace this lost fluid. Some older people have had surgery and a piece of small or large bowel is brought to the surface of the abdomen. This opening is known as a stoma. Faeces are collected in a bag which is attached to the abdominal wall. One of the functions of the large bowel (which is known as the colon) is to reabsorb water from faeces. People who have stomas may have either ileostomies (where the small bowel – known as the ileum – is brought to the surface of the abdomen) or colostomies (where a piece of the large bowel is brought to the surface of the abdomen). People who have stomas lose more fluid in their faeces than normal. People who have ileostomies tend to lose much more fluid than those who have colostomies. Individuals who are losing more fluid than average in their faeces must drink extra fluids to make up for the loss.

Older people, especially women, are more likely to develop cystitis and urine infections. These are normally treated with antibiotics but an important part of treating urine infections is encouraging the individual to drink lots of fluid. This helps flush the infection out of the system.

Normally healthy people breathe in and out through the nose. The breathing rate (known as the respiration rate) varies from 12 to 20 times per minute in healthy adults. If the older person develops a heavy cold or a chest infection, the nose can become blocked and the individual breathes through the mouth. The mouth then becomes dry and the amount of fluid lost in breathing is increased. The respiration rate increases when an individual develops a chest infection and the amount of fluid lost in breathing increases. A high temperature will normally develop and this will lead to increased sweating and more fluid will be required.

Helping and encouraging older people to drink

Before the carer can encourage the older person to drink she needs to find out what fluids the older person prefers. There is no point in offering the individual tea four times each day if she detests tea and relishes coffee. The carer should find out which fluids the individual prefers. Does the patient like tea? Does she like it black, with lemon, strong or weak? If the older person prefers sweet tea and cannot have sugar because she has diabetes, it is worth checking which sweetener is preferred. Some can leave a bitter after-taste. If the individual likes sugar in her tea don't forget to stir the tea or provide a teaspoon, otherwise all the sugar stays in the bottom of the cup, the tea tastes bitter and the person may not drink it.

If the individual likes coffee find out how he likes it. He may not appreciate mellow powdered coffee and may long for a rich, darkly roasted coffee. On the other hand he may detest the pungent, almost black coffee offered and prefer coffee made with milk and two sugars.

What cold drinks does the patient prefer? Not everyone likes orange squash. Some people may prefer orange barley water, fresh orange juice, lime juice, blackcurrant squash, apple juice or fruits of the forest. Some people may prefer fizzy drinks and may like lemonade, ginger beer, cola or even fizzy water. Low calorie still and fizzy drinks are available for people who are diabetic or who are trying to lose a little weight.

The individual may like to have a can of beer in the evening. Carers should check with professional staff before suggesting that the older person can have alcohol as some medicines react with alcohol and increase the risk of unpleasant side effects. Drinks should be served at the right temperature. Orange squash made with cold water is much more appealing than squash made with lukewarm water. Squashes should not be overdiluted as they then look unappealing and have no taste at all. Tea and coffee should be served hot, not lukewarm. Carers, though, should make sure that tea and coffee is not so hot that it could burn the mouth of a confused patient, or scald someone who accidentally spills the drink onto their lap.

If the older person has difficulty in communicating or is confused, family and friends can often advise staff on the individual's preferences. Staff should make a record of these preferences so that all staff can offer preferred fluids.

Some older people may not drink because the carer has left a jug of orange but has not left a glass. Sometimes the carer is aware that the patient does not have a drinking glass, means to bring it later but forgets. Many older people worry about being thought of as 'a nuisance' and do not wish to 'trouble the staff when they are busy'. If the older person does not have a glass she may remain thirsty for hours. Sometimes the drink is left just out of the older person's reach. Some older people can become forgetful and may forget to have the drink which has been poured and left; popping back to remind the older person only takes a moment and can prevent dehydration. Some older people cannot manage to lift heavy pottery cups full of tea. Providing lightweight cups such as those used on picnics can mean that the individual can drink independently. These cups look and feel just like normal cups. The patient or her family could choose lightweight cups if the home does not provide them.

It is almost impossible to drink if you are slumped in a chair or lying in bed. It is important that the carer helps the older person sit up comfortably so that she is able to drink. Some patients may have problems swallowing, especially those who have suffered from strokes or who have Parkinson's disease or motor neurone disease. Many of these individuals will require help to sit up and drink. If a patient appears to be choking on a drink the carer should stop giving the drink immediately and seek professional advice. Details of how to cope in an emergency are given in Chapter 6.

Giving fluids to frail people

Some older people are unable to drink fluids and rely on carers to give fluids. In many homes it is assumed that if the patient requires help a feeding cup should be used. Feeding cups are usually made of opaque white plastic and have a top with a spout on them.

Many older people manage to drink from a normal cup if the carer holds it to the patient's lips. It is important not to fill the cup too full and to take time helping the patient to drink. Some older people manage to drink cold fluids more easily using a flexible straw which bends over. If this is not possible, the carer may have no choice but to use a feeding cup, but these should not be used if there is an alternative. Feeding cups give patients very little control over how fast they drink. It can be easy to give the patient mouthfuls which are too large to swallow comfortably. Ask one of your colleagues to give you some tea from a tea cup. Now ask to be given tea in a feeding cup. Did you feel more in control when drinking from the cup? Which drink was more enjoyable.

Carers must always remember to ensure that they offer frail older people the fluids they prefer. Some people do not like to drink a great deal of fluid at once. The carer should respect the older person's wishes and offer 'little and often' in such a situation

Recording fluid intake and output

Professional staff may decide that an individual's fluid intake and output should be recorded. There are a number of reasons for this. Staff may be unsure how much the individual is drinking. Recording the amount allows staff to check if the person is drinking enough. Sometimes an individual is not drinking enough and all staff are asked to encourage and help the person to have sufficient fluids. The chart allows staff to check how successful they are in giving the person fluids. In other cases staff may be interested in how often the person in passing urine and how much is passed. This information is used to help people who have problems with incontinence. Further details on this are given in Chapter 13. Fluid charts are also called fluid balance charts. An example is given in Fig. 12.1.

Fluid charts are normally commenced at midnight. Some have continuous or running totals whilst others are added up at midnight. All fluid taken into the body is recorded on the left hand side of the chart. This includes not only fluids drunk but also fluid given by an intravenous infusion (drip) or directly into the stomach using either a tube which goes from the patient's nose (nasogastric tube) or one that is stitched into the patient's stomach (gastrostomy tube). Trained staff in nursing homes will record fluids given

Fluid Balance Chart

Name _____ Date _____

Time	Fluid type/amount	R/T	Output type/amount	R/T
	Total intake =		Total output =	

Fig. 12.1   Fluid balance chart.

intravenously or via gastrostomy or nasogastric tubes. Residential homes do not care for older people who require these types of feeding.

The right hand side of the chart is used to record fluids which leave the body. Urine is measured and recorded. If the patient vomits the amount of vomit is usually estimated and recorded on this side of the chart.

It is important to record fluids as accurately as possible. Carers may be asked to record fluids which patients have drunk on the fluid balance chart. Senior staff will show you how to do this.

The importance of a healthy diet

Older people require the same amount of vitamins and nutrients as younger people, according to Department of Health guidance. On average, though, older people require fewer calories than younger, more active people. Food provided to older people living in homes needs to be carefully selected. It should be as full of vitamins and nutrients as possible but should have fewer calories than our normal diet. A healthy diet makes the person feel well and protects against infection and illness.

How many calories does an older person require?

The amount of calories required varies from person to person. The active, older person living in a residential home, who is fairly independent, will normally require more calories than the person who lives in a nursing home who is not active. The inactive person living in a nursing home may, however, sometimes require more calories than the average older person. If the patient is recovering from a major operation, such as repair of a fractured femur, a diet high in calories, protein and vitamins will be required. If the patient has a wound, for example a pressure sore, extra calories, vitamins and protein are required in order to enable the wound to heal.

Some people living in homes will require large portions of food to meet their requirements, whilst others must avoid eating too much if they are to avoid gaining a great deal of weight. Weighing individuals from time to time will warn staff if the person is not having enough food or is gaining weight rapidly. In many hospitals all elderly people are weighed each week. If the older person is not seriously undernourished, monthly weighings are adequate.

What is a healthy diet?

Over the years, experts have given different and contradictory advice about a healthy diet. No doubt this advice will change again as experts learn more about nutrition. The Department of Health issues dietary guidelines for healthy eating, but these do not apply to elderly people. The guidelines, for example, recommend that adults should drink skimmed milk instead of whole milk, should reduce the amount of fat in their diets, should eat only two or three eggs per week, and should eat cheeses low in fat instead of high fat cheeses such as cheddar. But these recommendations are not suitable for elderly people, who require a diet full of vitamins and nutrients and containing a balance of protein, fat and carbohydrate.

Protein
Protein is found in meat, fish, nuts, lentils and beans. Protein is required to repair and replace tissues. People who have wounds, who have had recent surgery or who are recovering from a major illness require higher than normal amounts of protein.

Carbohydrate

Carbohydrate is found in vegetables and cereals. Carbohydrate is required to provide energy. It is converted by the body into glucose. Glucose is the body's main source of energy and is required by every living cell.

Fat
Fat is found in meat, fish, nuts, butter, margarine, cheese, eggs and cream. Fat is required to provide energy.

Vitamins and minerals

All food contains vitamins and minerals. Each vitamin and mineral has a function, and a shortage of vitamins or minerals can lead to illness. Some minerals and vitamins are found in most food, and shortage is rare. Others are only contained in a limited range of foods and if the individual does not eat these foods he may lack these vitamins or minerals.

The minerals and salts required by the body are given here.

Calcium

Calcium is found in milk, butter and cheese and in other foods. Calcium is required to maintain healthy teeth and bones. It also affects blood clotting and enables nerve cells to pass messages to each other. Older people can become short of calcium because they do not eat enough dairy produce. Vitamin D is required to enable the body to absorb calcium.

Copper and cobalt

Shortage of these minerals is very rare.

Iodine

Iodine is normally contained in the soil and vegetables grown in such soil absorb it. Sea fish and shell fish are a rich source of iodine.

Most people living in homes eat sea fish at least once a week and are not at risk of iodine deficiency. Even those who do not eat fish get enough iodine from fruit and vegetables.

Iron

Iron is found in red meat, beef, spinach, broccoli, apricots and chocolate. Many older people suffer from iron deficiency. This may be because they find it difficult to chew red meat, because they do not eat enough foods containing iron or because they have lost blood following an operation.

Some tablets, especially those given to people who suffer from arthritis – the anti-inflammatory drugs – can irritate the lining of the stomach and bowel. This irritation can cause the stomach and bowel to bleed a little, and this slow bleeding can cause the older person to develop anaemia. Iron tablets are usually given to treat anaemia. Only one tenth of iron in the diet or given in tablet form is normally absorbed by the body. If the person is anaemic the body absorbs more of the iron given. It has been found that the body can absorb more iron if vitamin C is given at the same time. Giving the older person an orange to eat or a glass of orange juice after iron tablets helps the body to absorb the iron.

Magnesium
Lack of magnesium is rare.

Sodium
This is normal salt. Fruit and vegetables contain salt. Most people add salt to their food and a shortage of salt is rare in this country. In tropical countries individuals may need to take extra salt on their food if they are working very hard and losing salt in their sweat.

Phosphorus
Phosphorus is found in milk, eggs and butter. It is needed to help muscles work properly, to form bones and to balance the chemicals in the body known as electrolytes. Shortage is very rare.

Zinc
This mineral is required to allow wounds and bones to heal. It is found in liver, eggs, meat and bran. Research in recent years has shown that some people who have wounds which fail to heal, such as pressure sores and leg ulcers, benefit from zinc supplements.

Vitamin A
Vitamin A is found in milk, butter, cream, eggs, liver, carrots and spinach. It is added to margarine. It is required to keep the skin and eyes healthy. Recent research suggests that vitamin A helps to protect the body against developing cancer.

Vitamin B
Vitamin B complex is really a series of vitamins.
Folic acid is found in green leafy vegetables, liver, yeast, Marmite (which is made from yeast) and beer. Shortage of folic acid causes anaemia. Some people who are suffering from anaemia are treated with a mixture of iron (ferrous sulphate) and folic acid.
Niacin is found in cereals, wheat, liver, yeast and fish. Deficiency is usually only found in countries where wheat flour is not eaten, but it can occur in alcoholics. Deficiency causes a disease known as pellagra and the person affected suffers from confusion, dementia, diarrhoea and dermatitis. Pellagra is very rare in the UK.
Thiamine is found in eggs, peas, beans, nuts, yeast, liver, kidneys and the outer husk of rice. Deficiency leads to a disease known as beri beri which is very rare in this country as thiamine is found in such a variety of foods.
Riboflavin is found in green vegetables, milk, cheese, eggs, yeast and liver. It is needed to maintain a healthy skin. Deficiency is rare and normally only occurs in people who for medical reasons have been taking antibiotics for a long period.

Vitamin B$_{12}$ is found in meat, especially liver and kidneys. Deficiency causes a special type of anaemia known as pernicious anaemia. Some people are unable to absorb vitamin B$_{12}$ because their stomach lacks a substance necessary to absorb it. People who suffer from vitamin B$_{12}$ deficiency have injections of this vitamin, given monthly or less frequently. Vegetarians can suffer from a shortage of vitamin B$_{12}$ but eating foods containing yeast, such as Marmite, or drinking beer (in moderation) can prevent this.

Vitamin C
Vitamin C is required to maintain a healthy skin and to enable wounds to heal. It is thought that vitamin C protects the body against infection. Fresh fruit and vegetables contain vitamin C. Citrus fruits are high in vitamin C, while apples, pears and plums contain only small amounts. Vitamin C is easily destroyed by cooking, and keeping vegetables warm (for example in a hot trolley) destroys the vitamin C content.

Vitamin D
Vitamin D is required to produce and maintain strong bones. Oily fish such as herrings, salmon and tuna, butter, margarine, cheese, eggs and liver contain vitamin D. The body can also make vitamin D. Spending half an hour, even in winter, outside with the hands and face exposed to sunlight enables the body to make enough vitamin D for its needs. Elderly people who are housebound and who have a poor diet may develop vitamin D deficiency. People with dark skins are more at risk of developing vitamin D deficiency in this country. Women who cover their hands and face, such as Muslim women, are at risk of developing vitamin D deficiency.

Vitamin K
Vitamin K is required to enable blood to clot normally. Vitamin K is found in meat and green vegetables. It is also produced by the body in the small intestine. Deficiency is rare.

Special diets

Some older people living in homes require special diets.

Diabetic diet
Older people who suffer from diabetes require a special diet. Normally when we eat, the pancreas produces insulin. Insulin enables us to use the glucose which is produced when food is digested. People who suffer from diabetes either do not produce any insulin or do not produce enough insulin.

There are two different types of diabetes. Type one usually occurs when the person is young. It is treated with insulin injections and a diabetic diet. Type two diabetes is also known as maturity onset diabetes; the pancreas fails to produce enough insulin for the person's needs. This form of diabetes is less severe than type one diabetes and can sometimes be treated with diet alone. Many people who suffer from type two diabetes are overweight and losing weight helps to control the disease. Some older people are given tablets. These tablets make the pancreas work harder to produce insulin and a combination of tablets and a diabetic diet is used to control diabetes.

Diabetes becomes more common as people age. Research has shown that by the age of 85 one tenth of all older people suffer from diabetes. Some people are more at risk of diabetes than others. Research shows that Asian people are more likely to become diabetic than other races. The reasons for this are not known.

The aim of a diabetic diet is to provide a diet high in fibre and low in fat and sugar. Fresh vegetables and fruit are recommended. The diabetic person can eat starchy foods such as potatoes, but baked potatoes are preferable to chips as they contain more fibre and less fat. The diabetic person should avoid sugar and sweet foods. Diabetics can eat sugar-free puddings. Many desserts are now available which use artificial sweeteners instead of sugar and these are suitable for diabetics. Special biscuits, sweets, chocolates, marmalade and jam can be bought for diabetics.

Overweight diabetics should avoid eating too many 'diabetic' foods. These are sweetened using a substance called sorbitol which is just as fattening as sugar. Too much sorbitol can cause diarrhoea; a diabetic person who eats a whole packet of sugar free mints or a packet of diabetic custard creams may suffer from acute diarrhoea. Tea and coffee can be sweetened with artificial sweeteners. An artificial sweetener which looks like sugar can be sprinkled over cereals, used to sweeten custard and used instead of sugar in cakes.

Reducing diets

Reducing diets are intended to help overweight people lose weight. Being overweight can make an older person unwell, and losing weight can make them feel better. People who have high blood pressure who are overweight may find that their blood pressure improves if they lose weight. People who suffer from arthritis, especially arthritis of the hips and knees, place an extra strain on joints if they are overweight. Losing weight can help reduce pain and increase movement.

The aim of a reducing diet is to produce a small, steady loss in weight. It is important that the older person has a diet with sufficient vitamins and nutrients. Usually the amount of sugar in the diet is reduced. Sweeteners can be used in tea and coffee and on cereals. Fat can be reduced: the older person can have grilled bacon instead of fried, a poached egg instead of a fried egg. Occasional treats such as cake or a small bar of chocolate should be allowed, otherwise the person who is on a reducing diet may decide to give up. If the older person is overweight and does not wish to lose weight, staff working in the home must respect the person's wishes.

Vegetarians

Vegetarians do not eat meat. Some vegetarians eat fish, eggs and dairy products whilst others do not eat any animal products. People who do not eat any animal products are known as vegans. It is important to ensure that people who are vegetarian are offered a healthy vegetarian diet. Details on obtaining information on vegetarian diets appear in the further information section at the end of the chapter.

High fibre diets

High fibre diets help prevent constipation. Further details on the reasons why older people are at risk of developing constipation are given in Chapter 13. A diet rich in fibre can enable older people to have normal bowel actions and avoid relying on laxatives.

There are two different types of fibre: soluble and non-soluble. It is recommended that a high fibre diet should contain a mixture of both types. This means that the diet should contain fruit and vegetables and also fibre found in cereals such as porridge, Weetabix, All bran, wholemeal bread, digestive biscuits and wholemeal flour.

A high fibre diet can be tasty and varied but should be introduced gradually so that the person's body can get used to it. All people are different and the amount of fibre people require varies. One person may find that the diet provides too much fibre and causes diarrhoea, whilst another might require extra fibre perhaps by having an extra portion of fruit, a dish of prunes or a slice of date loaf.

High calorie diet

High calorie diets are required when the older person is thin and undernourished or has increased dietary needs, perhaps because he is more active than other patients, is recovering from a recent operation or has a pressure sore or leg ulcer. The aim is to provide enough calories to meet the patient's needs. Putting too much food on the plate can be off-putting so carers should offer snacks, encourage family and friends to bring in foods which the person is especially fond of, and give dietary supplements if they have been supplied by the doctor.

Puréed diets

Some older people who are very frail or who have difficulty in chewing, perhaps because of a stroke, may require a puréed diet. The aim is to give, as far as possible, a normal diet which has been puréed. Meat and vegetables should not be mixed together and puréed as this is unappetising and the person cannot choose which part of the meal to eat. Food should be puréed separately and served in a dish with partitions so that the different foods do not blend into each other. The person receiving a puréed diet may also require dietary supplements.

Meeting the dietary needs of people from different cultures

Some older people come from different backgrounds to those of the majority of people living in homes. People who come from different cultures or who practice different religions may require a different diet. The aim of care in homes is to provide a similar type of life to that which the person would lead living at home. Research shows that although there are a significant number of people from different cultures living in the UK, few people from ethnic minorities enter homes. The reasons for this are not known but there are several theories.

Many people come to the UK from other countries when they are young. In the 1950s many people came to the UK from the West Indies. They were recruited by London transport to work on the railways, tubes and buses. Since then many younger people have entered the UK from other countries. People who came to the UK in the 1950s are only just becoming old and may require care in homes.

Another theory is that already many people from other cultures require care in homes but because homes do not provide special services to meet their needs they are reluctant to enter homes. It is important that all older people living in homes have their needs met and their cultures respected.

People from different cultures have different dietary needs.

Jewish

Jewish people eat a special diet which is called a *kosher* diet. Those who follow this diet strictly have separate areas within the kitchen for preparing meat and milk dishes. Milk and meat are not eaten together and separate crockery is used for meat and milk dishes. Even people of the Jewish faith who do not have a strict kosher diet normally avoid having meat and milk at the same meal. The person may have cereal with milk for breakfast but would not eat a beef sausage at this meal. Jewish people do not normally eat pork or shellfish. There is a special nursing home in London for Jewish people and a strict kosher diet is available in the home. If a carer is caring for a person of the Jewish faith she should find out what the person prefers to eat and drink.

Muslims

Muslims do not eat pork and normally avoid alocohol. Strict Muslims eat meat which has been killed in a special way, known as *halal* meat. This can be obtained from halal butchers and is cooked normally. If halal meat is not available strict Muslims may prefer to avoid eating meat.

Hindus

Hindus do not eat beef. Some people of the Hindu faith are completely vegetarian and do not eat any animal products.

Dietary supplements

Older people who are unable to eat enough food to meet their requirements are often offered dietary supplements. There is an enormous range of dietary supplements available. These include drinks which look and taste like squash but are high in calories, vitamins and minerals. Other drinks are like milk shakes and come in a range of flavours; these too are full of vitamins, minerals and calories. Special puddings are available, and special high protein snacks such as biscuits may also be given.

If the older person appears to be losing weight or is not eating very much, professional advice should be sought. In nursing homes carers will be working under the supervision of trained nurses who will take appropriate action. In residential homes carers should ask the doctor to contact the dietician who will visit the patient. The dietician will normally bring a range of dietary supplements. The older person can taste these supplements and the dietician will normally contact the patient's doctors and ask for them to be prescribed. Dietary supplements are available on prescription to individuals who have difficulty in swallowing or who suffer from certain conditions.

Why some older people have difficulty eating

Chewing

Chewing can be difficult for some older people. Those who have lost their dentures or who have poorly fitting dentures will have difficulty. People who have suffered from strokes sometimes have difficulty in chewing because one side of the face is paralysed. Confused patients, especially those in the advanced stages of dementia, may not be aware that they are supposed to chew food and may leave the food sitting in the mouth unchewed.

Swallowing

Swallowing can be difficult. People who suffer from motor neurone disease, multiple sclerosis, Parkinson's disease or who have suffered from strokes may have difficulty in swallowing. Carers should encourage them to take small mouthfuls, chew thoroughly and wash food down well with water. The person who has difficulty in swallowing should sit up straight in the chair, as slouching makes the problem worse.

Cutlery

Cutlery can be difficult for some older people to use. The person who has lost the use of one hand may find it very difficult to cut up food and eat one-handed. Special cutlery is available to help people who can only use one hand. People who have severe arthritis in the hands can find it difficult to grip ordinary cutlery, and special cutlery is available for them.

Some people find that the plate slips. Non-slip mats placed under the plate prevent this. If a person is eating one-handed the food can easily slip off the plate. Using a plate guard which clips onto the plate prevents this. Aids to help older people to eat can be purchased from medical supplies companies or they can be supplied by the occupational therapist for the individual's use. The patient's doctor can ask the occupational therapist to visit to provide suitable aids.

Poor eyesight

Poor eyesight can prevent people from seeing the food on the plate. Using dark coloured plates to provide a contrast enables the older person to see the food more easily.

Confused patients

Confused patients can find it difficult to settle down to eat a meal. Creating a relaxed, calm atmosphere helps confused patients to settle and enjoy their meal. Turning off the television, playing music and avoiding bustling about help to create a relaxing meal time.

Making meal times a pleasure

Mealtimes should be pleasant occasions and should give the older person the opportunity not only to enjoy a meal but also to chat with others and to relax over the meal (Fig. 12.2). It is important that staff make a little effort to make eating a pleasant experience. In many nursing homes breakfast is served in the patient's room. The older person should be made comfortable for breakfast and helped to sit up in bed or to sit out in a chair if she requires help. Food should be presented attractively and served hot. Lukewarm tea and cold porridge do not encourage people to eat.

Many homes encourage older people to eat lunch in the dining room so that they can chat with others. Tables should be set out with table cloths, napkins, cutlery, drinks, salt, pepper and sauces. Older people who are able to help lay tables should be encouraged to do so. Playing music quietly in the background helps create a relaxing atmosphere and encourages people to relax and enjoy their meal. People who require help with feeding can be helped by carers. Carers should sit with the individual who requires help, as this makes the person feel more relaxed and less hurried.

Fig. 12.2   A group of patients enjoying their lunch.

Summary

Eating and drinking are essential if the individual is to remain in good health. Some older people living in homes require help to eat and drink; others, especially those with special dietary needs, may require advice on what foods they should eat. Carers should be aware of the older person's fluid and food preferences. Carers should aim to provide, wherever possible, food and drink which the older person prefers. The food available should be similar to that which the older person would choose to eat at home. Carers should offer to assist older people who require help and should be careful to ensure that the older person maintains dignity at all times.

Portfolio preparation

- Identify individuals within your home who have difficulty eating and drinking. How are they helped to overcome these difficulties?
- Ask if you can take copies of their care plans. Remember to remove the person's name to protect confidentiality.
- Find out what aids are available within the home to help individuals retain the ability to eat and drink independently.
- Find out if any of the patients in the home have a special diet for medical reasons, for example a diabetic diet. Include details and a copy of a diet sheet for an individual with diabetes in your portfolio.
- If any of the patients come from different cultures and require a special diet, gives details of that diet and explain how it is offered within the home.

Further information

The British Diabetic Association (BDA)
10 Queen Anne Street
London W1M 0BD
Telephone 0171 323 1531

Further information on all aspects of diabetes and diabetic diets is available from the BDA. They produce a range of leaflets, books and videos and will send a catalogue on request.

Vegetarian Society
Dale Park
Durham Road
Altringham
Cheshire
WA14 4QG
Telephone 0161 928 0793.

Further information on vegetarian diets is available from the Vegetarian Society. They produce a useful leaflet *Healthy Nutrition in Later Life*, which contains guidance and recipes and is available free if an SAE is sent.

Kelloggs Education Pack
Freepost
Horndean
Waterlooville
Hants PO8 9BR.

Further information on high fibre diets is available from Kelloggs. They produce a patient education pack and a selection of recipes.

Chapter 13

Promotion of Continence

Introduction

> This chapter will give information on the normal functions of the bladder and bowel. Information given in this chapter includes:
>
> - understanding elimination
> - how ageing affects bladder function
> - enabling older people to use the toilet independently
> - dignity and privacy
> - health and safety
> - continence problems, including overactive bladder, stress and overflow incontinence
> - how medicines, mobility and mental state affect continence
> - continence promotion – bladder re-training and timed voiding
> - incontinence pads
> - catheters and penile sheaths
> - bowel care
> - constipation
> - diarrhoea
> - stoma care
> - disposing of body waste

Understanding elimination

The kidneys produce urine, and in doing so carry out three functions:

- removing waste products from the blood
- conserving water and salt
- maintaining the balance of chemicals in the blood (electrolyte balance)

The amount of urine produced varies depending on the amount of fluid the person has consumed and the amount of fluid lost. On a very hot day, if the person does not drink extra fluid, the urine will become more concentrated. The kidneys concentrate the urine to maintain the balance of fluid within the body. If the person drinks a lot, more urine is produced. Many people notice that they pass more urine in cold water; this is because less fluid is lost through sweating so urine production is increased to maintain the balance of fluid within the body. The average person drinking two litres of fluid each day will produce about 1500 ml of urine each day. Most urine is formed when we are awake; at night a hormone is produced which enables the kidneys to concentrate urine. This hormone is known as anti-diuretic hormone. The colour of urine varies according to how concentrated it is. Normally the urine passed first thing in the morning is darker because it is more concentrated. Urine is normally yellow or straw coloured.

Urine drains from the kidneys into the ureters (Fig. 13.1). It is then collected in the bladder. The bladder is a little like a balloon. It stretches in all directions to allow it to fill with urine and contracts in all directions to empty. The bladder contains special nerves known as stretch receptors. These send a message to the brain when the bladder is becoming full.

The amount of urine the bladder holds varies; the male bladder

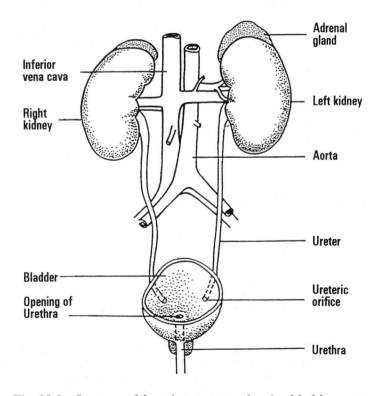

Fig. 13.1 Anatomy of the urinary system showing bladder, ureters and urethra.

can hold more than the female and some people have larger bladders than others. The urethra drains urine from the bladder.

How ageing affects the function of the kidneys and bladder

The kidneys work less efficiently in older people. They become less efficient at concentrating urine, so older people become dehydrated more easily than younger people. Older people usually produce more urine at night because of this. It is quite normal for an older person to have to get up once or twice in the night to pass urine. This is because the bladder becomes smaller in old age and less stretchy, and can hold less urine. When we pass urine a small amount is left in the bladder; this is known as residual urine. As people age and the bladder is less able to push urine out, the amount of urine left in the bladder increases.

Men have a gland known as the prostate gland, shown in Fig. 13.2. This enlarges with age and can make it more difficult for the bladder to empty completely. Women (Fig. 13.3) produce female hormones called oestrogen and progesterone. Hormone production is greatly reduced after the menopause and sometimes lack of oestrogen can lead to incontinence.

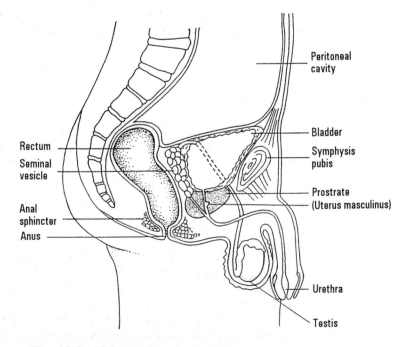

Fig. 13.2   Male genito-urinary tract.

Fig. 13.3   Female genito-urinary tract.

As people age the special nerves in the bladder (stretch receptors), which warn that the bladder is becoming full, become less sensitive. Adults are aware of the sensation of bladder fullness when the bladder is 50% full. The older person is not normally aware of the sensation of bladder fullness until the bladder is 90% full.

Examining and testing urine

Normal urine is clear. Urine which is cloudy or thick or has bits floating in it should be saved and professional advice sought. Fresh urine does not smell. Urine which has been standing or which has been collecting in a catheter bag may smell because bacteria break down urine and produce ammonia. Urine should be golden or straw coloured. The first specimen of the day is usually darker. Dark urine is more concentrated than light urine and is normally a sign that the individual is not drinking enough. Some drugs and foods can cause the urine to change colour. Eating beetroot can produce red or pink urine. Some people who are prescribed the antibiotic nitofuridantoin produce turquoise urine. If the urine is not the normal colour carers should save the specimen and seek professional advice. Blood may cause the urine to appear red or pink. If the carer suspects that the urine contains blood, professional advice should be obtained immediately.

Urine is normally tested when an older person is admitted to the home. Testing urine enables staff to detect abnormalities. Urine is normally tested with a Multi-stick. This is a plastic strip which has a number of pads on it. Each pad has chemicals on it and changes colour when it is dipped in fresh urine and an abnormality is present. Urine is normally checked for a number of substances.

Blood
Blood in the urine can be caused by infection, kidney stones or other conditions.

Ketones
Ketones are substances produced when the body is burning up fat. This occurs if the person is diabetic and the diabetes is poorly controlled. Ketones are also present in the urine of people who are losing weight. The overweight person who is on a diet may have ketones in the urine. Undernourished people and people who have been vomiting (and are therefore not eating) may have ketones in their urine.

Glucose
Glucose or sugar may be present in the urine of people who have diabetes.

Protein
Protein may be present in the urine of people who have kidney disease or who have a urine infection.

pH
pH indicates if the urine is acid or alkaline. The pH of urine is normally between five and seven. A pH above seven may indicate that the person has an infection. Vegetarians normally have a urine pH of above seven and this is normal for people who do not eat meat.

Some urine testing sticks also measure the *specific gravity*. This enables staff to check how concentrated urine is. The normal specific gravity of urine is 1002 to 1030. A specific gravity of more than 1030 indicates that the urine is very concentrated. Some sticks also test for *nitrite*. Nitrite is produced when an infection is present.

Urine test sticks will give inaccurate results if they are not stored properly. It is important to close the container tightly and not to remove the small packet which is in the bottle with the sticks. The packet contains crystals which prevent the sticks becoming damp and giving a false reading.

Faeces

Faeces contain waste products and food such as fibre which cannot be digested by the body. Faeces are normally brown and soft. Bile salts give faeces their brown colour. The normal stool is produced without straining. The amount of faeces produced varies according to how much fibre is eaten but between 80 and 200 g are produced each day. It normally takes three days for food to pass through the body. Bowel habits vary from individual to individual but research on large numbers of people shows that the normal range of bowel actions varies from three times per day to once every third day.

Some drugs can alter the appearance of faeces. Iron tablets cause the faeces to become black, sticky and look like tar. Some drugs can cause the individual to bleed either from the stomach or the bowel. Blood in faeces can also make them appear black and tar-like. If the individual bleeds from the lower bowel, blood can be seen clearly. Carers who see faeces which appear abnormal should save the specimen and obtain professional advice.

Enabling older people to use the toilet

Some older people living in homes will have difficulty walking. Often with help, encouragement, physiotherapy and walking aids they can regain the ability to walk to the toilet independently. Details on mobility are given in Chapter 8.

Some older people may have difficulty in identifying the toilets. If the toilets are in a corridor and all the doors look the same, it can be difficult to find the toilet. The older person with poor eyesight may be unable to read the small signs that say 'Toilet'. In some homes all toilet doors have been painted a special colour, perhaps yellow, so that they stand out from all the other doors. In other homes staff have made up large posters with pictures of toilets on them. Other homes have large signs saying 'Toilet' in letters six inches high. These measures help older people to find toilets quickly and enable them to use the toilet independently.

Some older men who have poor eyesight find it difficult to see the toilet. If the toilet and the floor are the same colour a poorly sighted man can find this difficult. In some homes a toilet seat in a contrasting colour such as black on a white toilet helps the patient to see the toilet. This method works unless the male patient is in the habit of lifting the toilet seat, as many men do. In some homes a coloured toilet cleanser is put in the cistern; each time the toilet is flushed it refills with blue coloured water. The poorly sighted male patient can then aim for the blue water.

Some patients who suffer from arthritis, especially arthritis of the hips and knees, can manage to sit on the toilet but find it difficult to get up because the seat is too low. Providing raised toilet seats which fit over the toilet can help arthritis patients to use the toilet independently.

Some patients may find it difficult to pull down or adjust clothing without help. Carers can suggest clothing which is easier to remove and adjust. Trousers with elastic waistbands are easier to manage than those with zips and buttons. Some male patients find jogging pants comfortable, but these seldom have zips in the front. Placing a zip in the front helps male patients to use the toilet without help. Some men's trousers have short zips; if these are replaced with longer zips many male patients find it easier to use the toilet.

Female patients may have difficulty pulling up dresses or skirts which are tightly fitted around the legs and hips. Wearing skirts and dresses which are flared or have pleats makes it easier to hitch up clothing and use the toilet.

Male and female patients should be advised to wear pants which are not too tight. Tight pants are not only uncomfortable but are difficult to pull down. Patients who have difficulty dressing and undressing can be encouraged to practice. There are many ways of learning to dress and undress which take disability into account. Further details are given in *All Dressed Up*, the book mentioned under Further Reading in the Clothing section of Chapter 11.

Some older people become forgetful and may lose track of time. Carers can help by reminding them to use the toilet. Reminding them first thing in the morning, before meals and in the evening may help the older person to remain continent.

Dignity and privacy

Using the toilet is a private activity. Older people who are using the toilet should be able to do so without fearing that carers or other patients will burst in on them. Toilets should have locks and older people should be encouraged to lock the toilet door. If the older person is using a commode or bedpan, perhaps in a shared bedroom, the bed curtains should be drawn to protect the individual's privacy and dignity. Does your home have a policy on privacy and dignity?

Health and safety

Although the older person has the right to privacy and dignity when using the toilet, staff may need to enter the toilet in the case of an emergency. The individual may have fallen or collapsed and requires urgent help. Many homes have toilets which can be opened by staff in an emergency. Some homes have doors which open if the edge of a coin is inserted in a slot on the outside of the door, and turned. Other homes use a master key system; the key is placed in the outside of the lock and turned. Can the doors in your home be opened from the outside in an emergency?

Most toilets have vinyl floors. Many floors are made of special vinyl which is non-slip even when wet. There is a danger, though, that people will slip over if walking on a wet floor. If the toilet floor is wet it should be cleaned and dried at once to prevent falls occurring.

Most toilets have special rails which older people can use to pull themselves up and hold onto when using the toilet. If these work lose, this should be reported at once and if possible the toilet should not be used until grab rails are made safe. If it is not possible to stop using the toilet, carers should accompany patients until repairs have been completed.

Older people who are using the toilet independently may require help. Toilets should have call bells fitted and these should be easily reached by patients.

Assisting older people to use toilets

Research has shown that people are more likely to suffer from incontinence if they have to depend on someone else to take them to the toilet. It is easy to understand the reasons for this. An older person asks the carer, 'Can you take me to the toilet please?'. The carer is busy laying the tables for lunch and says, 'Just a minute Mrs Johnstone, I'll just finish laying the table.' The carer finishes laying the table and helps Mrs Johnstone to the toilet. Mrs Johnstone walks very slowly because she has had a stroke, her balance is poor and she uses a tripod. The toilet is some distance away. Mrs Johnstone and the carer enter the toilet and while Mrs Johnstone is holding on to the grab rail so that the carer can pull down her pants, she wets herself.

The section on the effects of ageing on the bladder at the beginning of the chapter explained how older people have less warning about the need to empty their bladders than younger people. Mrs Johnstone only became aware of the need to use the toilet when her bladder was almost full. She may have noticed that the staff were busy and waited until it seemed convenient; by then she was bursting to go. The carer who is aware of how ageing and illness affect the bladder would have reacted differently. When Mrs Johnstone asked to go to the toilet the carer would have come over at once and asked, 'Are you desperate or have we got time to walk there?' Mrs Johnstone would have replied, 'No, I'm not desperate, we have plenty of time.' Because the carer responded promptly, Mrs Johnstone had plenty of time to walk to the toilet. Had her need been more urgent, the carer could have wheeled her to the toilet and walked her back. The episode of incontinence would have been avoided.

If the older person is desperate to use the toilet but staff are encouraging the person to walk, wheeling her to the toilet and helping her to walk back will help the person to exercise and provide sensitive care.

If older people require help to use the toilet, carers should help the person to sit on the toilet, ensure that the individual can reach the call bell and offer to wait outside. The older person can call when she has finished. It is important to help the older person to wash her hands after using the toilet. Carers should wash their hands each time they take an individual to the toilet. This is very important as it prevents the spread of infection.

Commodes

Commodes are sometimes used in homes. Often older people who need to use the toilet at night are helped on and off commodes. Bedcurtains should be used at all times.

Bedpans

Bedpans are sometimes offered when the individual is in bed. It can be very difficult to sit comfortably on a bedpan and some patients are unable to pass urine in them because they fear that the urine will splash on the bed. It is important that carers find out if the older person prefers to use a commode or a bedpan.

How the bladder works

We are all born incontinent (Fig. 13.4) but learn to control our bladders as young children. When the bladder fills with urine it begins to contract and the urethra which acts as a plug to hold urine in, relaxes. Urine is then forced out. When we develop control of our bladders a signal is sent to our brain when the bladder is almost full. The brain then sends a signal back to the bladder telling it to hold on. This signals acts by stopping the bladder from contracting and tightening up the urethra. We then hold on until we can find a toilet, adjust our clothes and pass urine.

This is demonstrated in Fig. 13.5. Normally people empty their bladders between four and eight times each day.

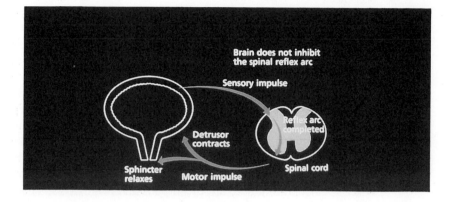

Fig. 13.4   How a baby's bladder works by simple spinal reflex arc.

Fig. 13.5   Adult bladder control. Nerve pathways between the bladder, spine and micturition control centre. (Note: the nerves supplying the urethra are not shown in the diagram.)

Continence problems

Incontinence is the inability to control bladder or bowels. Urinary incontinence, the inability to control the bladder, is much more common.

Most people feel that such a problem is shameful and are very embarrassed and upset by it. They fear that others may feel that they are dirty or lazy. Many older people who have problems controlling their bladders go to great lengths to conceal it. The older person living in a home may ask her family to bring in sanitary towels. She may use serviettes or toilet paper to line her pants. If her pants become wet she may wash them out and try to dry them on the radiator to prevent staff finding out.

Some staff working in homes, including some trained nurses, do not realise that many people who develop incontinence can be helped to become continent again. In some homes if a person becomes incontinent they are given pads and not treated. This is poor care. Incontinence is not a disease; it is a sign that something is wrong. It is often possible to discover and treat the problem causing the incontinence.

Continence assessments

Every person who has a continence problem should be seen and investigated. Professional staff who are qualified to carry out such investigations are:

- GPs
- District nurses
- Registered nurses

These staff may ask a nurse specially trained in helping people regain continence and in caring for incontinence. These nurses are known as continence advisers and have special training to help them work with people suffering from incontinence.

Causes of incontinence

There are many reasons why a person develops incontinence. Some of these are bladder problems but sometimes incontinence has other causes. The treatment given varies because the cause of incontinence is different in different patients.

Overactive bladder

This is sometimes known as urgency or urge incontinence. The technical term for urge incontinence is *bladder dysreflexia*. You may notice, or the patient may complain that:

- the person goes to the toilet very frequently and has to use the toilet more than twice each night
- the patient has to rush to get to the toilet – sometimes just as she gets to the toilet she wets on the floor
- she may sometimes wet the bed a little at night.

Causes

The bladder muscles start to contract before the bladder is completely full. The individual is unable to stop the muscle contracting down and hold on. Urgency affects older men and women and is a very common problem. Patients who have had strokes or who suffer from Parkinson's disease may find urgency a problem. In many cases the cause is still unknown. It is well known, though, that worry and nerves can make the bladder more likely to develop urgency. Some people find that when they are anxious they develop a headache or diarrhoea, whilst others find they keep needing to go to the toilet. If the older person is worried about wetting herself, this makes the situation worse.

Treatment

Urge incontinence is usually treated with bladder retraining. Details are given later in this chapter. In some cases drugs are also used.

Overflow incontinence

Carers may notice that:

- the person is always on the toilet
- the person is in there for ages
- the person has to strain to pass urine
- urine is passed in little dribbles rather than a strong stream
- the person may dribble urine in between going to the toilet
- only very small amounts of urine are passed although the person was desperate to go
- the individual complains that he or she has not been properly and the bladder still feels full.

Causes

A blockage is preventing the bladder from emptying properly. The person can only pass small amounts of urine. The bladder is full and the person can only pass the small amount of urine which is leaking or overflowing from the bladder. Overflow incontinence affects both men and women. It is commoner in men and can be caused by an enlarged prostate gland. Many people who have suffered from stokes or who have multiple sclerosis or motor neurone disease develop overflow incontinence. One of the commonest causes of overflow incontinence is constipation. A bowel full of faeces squeezes against the urethra and prevents urine draining.

Treatment

Treatment of overflow incontinence depends on the cause. Constipation is easily treated and effective bowel management will prevent it recurring. Men who are suffering from an enlarged prostate will be sent to see a consultant urologist who will decide on appropriate treatment. In some cases catheters are used to drain urine. Further details on catheter care are given later in the chapter.

Stress incontinence

Carers may notice or patients may complain that:

■ the bladder leaks when the individual coughs, sneezes or walks around

Causes

The bladder is supported by muscles known as the pelvic floor. These muscles can become weakened and support the bladder less effectively. Urine is held in the bladder and the urethra acts as a plug until it is convenient to pass urine. The urethra may become less effective in women after menopause due to a shortage of the hormone oestrogen. Stress incontinence normally affects women. Only men who have had surgery to the prostate gland may have problems with stress incontinence.

Treatment

Treatment will vary according to the cause. Weak muscles may be treated with pelvic floor exercises. If the muscles are very weak surgery to repair the muscles and lift them back in place may be carried out. Many older women who have other health problems are not well enough to have surgery. A special ring (known as a ring pessary) may be inserted by the doctor or nurse specialist to hold up the womb if it is dropping down and pressing on the bladder. Sometimes these rings are coated with the female hormone oestrogen as this can help treat stress incontinence. These are usually changed by a doctor or nurse specialist every year. Sometimes a cream containing the hormone oestrogen is prescribed by the doctor. This is applied to the genital region and helps treat women who suffer from stress incontinence.

Other factors which cause incontinence

Many problems which cause incontinence are not bladder problems. Often the older person has been managing to control his or her bladder until a change in circumstances tips the individual over the edge into incontinence. Many things can cause incontinence, including the attitude of carers. The commonest reasons older people develop continence problems are given below.

Moving to a new place

Often when the older person is to be admitted to the home, staff ask if the person has a continence problem. The answer is often no, yet when the person arrives at the home she is incontinent. Leaving their own home where a person has lived for many years and entering a residential or nursing home is a stressful experience. The older person is usually admitted from hospital and may dread entering the home. She may have been transferred from an acute ward to an elderly care ward and then finally to the home. This makes most older people anxious and worried and this can affect the bladder and cause incontinence. Helping the person settle into the home, making her feel welcome and providing sensitive care can help clear up the incontinence quickly. Further details are given in Chapter 5.

Medicines

Medicines can cause incontinence. They can act in a number of ways, either working directly on the bladder or affecting the person's general health.

Diuretics are usually called water tablets by patients. They act on the kidneys and lead to more urine being produced. Diuretics are given to treat heart failure, to lower blood pressure or to treat swollen legs. There are many different types of diuretics. Some act slowly and gently, causing a little more urine to be produced throughout the day. Others have a more drastic action and cause the kidneys to produce large amounts of urine for a few hours. Diuretics are usually given in the morning. This can cause problems if the older person requires help to go to the toilet as staff are busiest in the morning, and a delay in responding to the person's request for help can lead to incontinence.

Many older people living in homes have sleeping tablets every night. Sleeping tablets cause people to be less alert and more drowsy, not just at night but also during the day. They can lead to incontinence. Some older people are anxious and upset when they enter homes. Some are prescribed sedatives and these can cause the person to become less alert and to become incontinent.

Other medicines can also cause incontinence. A continence assessment by a trained professional will include checking the patient's medication. If medication is causing incontinence this may be discontinued or changed by the patient's doctor.

Difficulty with walking

The older person who is unable to use the toilet without help is more likely to suffer from incontinence. Chapter 8 gives details of how carers can help older people regain independence and Chapter 9 gives information on helping the older person to move. It is important that carers respond promptly to calls for help to use the toilet.

Confusion

The person who is confused or forgetful may have problems remembering to go to the toilet. Reminding the person to go to the toilet at set times often helps to prevent incontinence.

Infection

A bladder infection causes the bladder to become more irritable and the person who has a bladder infection usually needs to go to the toilet frequently and pass small amounts of urine. Bladder infections can cause the individual to become confused and this can lead to incontinence.

One of the first signs of a chest infection in elderly people can be confusion. Elderly people can become very ill if they are suffering from a chest infection. The individual may be unable to walk to the toilet and because of confusion may be unable to ask for the toilet. Coughing can lead to stress incontinence. Fortunately the incontinence normally vanishes when the person recovers from the infection.

How carers can help

Carers can help by informing professionals if the older person is developing a bladder problem. The continence assessment includes keeping a record of everything a person drinks and all urine passed. A fluid chart is used. The fluid chart is normally kept for a week. The registered nurse or continence adviser may then ask for a bladder chart to be used. A copy is shown in Fig. 13.6.

Each time the person passes urine in the toilet the left hand side

BLADDER CHART

Week commencing: Name:

Please tick in the **plain** column each time you pass urine

Please tick in the **shaded** column each time you are wet

Special instructions:

	Monday	Tuesday	Wednesday	Thursday	Friday	Saturday	Sunday
Midnight							
1am							
2							
3							
4							
5							
6							
7							
8							
9							
10							
11							
Noon							
1pm							
2							
3							
4							
5							
6							
7							
8							
9							
10							
11							
Totals							

BLADDER TRAINING PROGRAMME

In order to bring your bladder problem under control, you must learn to stretch your bladder. You can do this by trying to hold on as long as possible before passing water. Do not restrict your fluid intake. You should drink no more or less than you normally do.

On the back of this sheet is a bladder chart to help you monitor your progress - fill this in **every time you pass urine normally** and **every time you are wet**.

❏ Place a tick in the **shaded** column to the nearest hour when you leak urine, place a tick in the **plain** column when you pass urine normally.

❏ When you get the feeling that you want to pass urine **try to hold on for as long as possible**.

❏ At first this will be difficult, but as you persevere it will become easier.

❏ If you wake up at night with a full bladder it is best to go and empty it straight away, as holding on will only keep you awake.

❏ Sitting on a hard seat may help you to hold your water.

❏ Your doctor may have prescribed tablets to help you hold your water. Take these regularly as directed.

❏ You should aim to gradually reduce the frequency with which you pass urine to 5 or 6 times in 24 hours.

REMEMBER

You are attempting to stretch your bladder. Although you may find this difficult at first, with practice it will get easier. If you persevere, you will be surprised at what you can achieve.

Fig. 13.6   Bladder chart.

of the chart is ticked. Each time the person is wet the right hand side of the chart is ticked. The chart is used to monitor the person's progress and to help decide on further treatment. This will vary from person to person and will depend on the nature of the problem.

Bladder retraining

Bladder retraining is used to help patients who suffer from urgency and have overactive bladders. The bladder chart enables professionals to see how often the person can hold on between visits to the toilet. The individual is encouraged to hold on for an extra 15 minutes between each visit to the toilet. Every three days the time between visits is increased by 15 minutes. Gradually the bladder is able to hold more urine and the person learns to control bladder contractions. Eventually the older person should be able to visit the toilet every two or three hours. Sometimes drugs are given to help increase the amount of urine the bladder can hold and dampen down bladder contractions. These drugs are known as anticholinergics.

Timed voiding

People who are confused or forgetful often forget to go to the toilet or do not understand the messages they receive to tell them their bladder is full up. The bladder chart enables professionals to discover the times the confused person is normally wet. The person is taken to the toilet before the time of incontinence and encouraged to use the toilet. Using this method it is possible to help about two-thirds of all confused patients regain continence. Unfortunately about one-third do not have a regular pattern of passing urine and timed toileting is hit and miss.

Caring for incontinent patients

Some patients cannot be helped to regain continence. Incontinence may be caused by either a physical problem such as motor neurone disease or an enlarged prostate, or a mental problem such as dementia. The aim of care is to collect the urine, prevent the patient becoming smelly, sore or wet, protect the skin and ensure that the patient's dignity is maintained at all times.

Incontinence pads

Incontinence pads are used to collect urine. They normally have a plastic backing and are filled with cellulose pulp (Fig. 13.7). The superabsorbent pads contain granules which swell up and form a gel when wet. This gel locks the urine into the pad and helps keep the patient's skin dry. Many pads have a liner which draws urine away from the skin. Some pads have a wetness indicator in the

Fig. 13.7   Incontinence pad.

plastic outer covering of the pad. The wetness indicator changes colour when the pad needs changing. If the person has been incontinent of faeces, the pad should be changed immediately to maintain patient comfort and prevent skin problems.

Pads work more effectively and are less likely to leak if they are fitted closely to the body. Most pad manufacturers recommend that the patient wears a pair of specially designed briefs made of nylon to hold the pad in place (Figs 13.8 and 13.9).

How often should pads be changed?

This will vary from person to person and will depend on the amount of urine produced. Pads may be changed every two to four hours. Pads should not be left unchanged for longer than four hours or skin problems can occur. Details on caring for the skin of incontinent patients are given in Chapter 11.

Dribble pads

These are small pads which fit over the penis and collect small drips or dribbles. Their use can preserve the male patient's dignity, protect clothing and prevent odour.

Re-usable incontinence pads

It is now possible to buy pants with a built in washable incontinence pad. These small pads can absorb up to 80 ml of urine. Some female patients who suffer from slight stress incontinence prefer these to a pad. The pants are, of course, named and are the personal underwear of that particular patient. It is important not to use fabric conditioner on these pants as it prevents them absorbing urine.

Obtaining incontinence pads

At the moment people who suffer from incontinence and who are cared for in residential homes are issued with pads by the local NHS trust. If you work in a home run by social services these pads are delivered to the home. In most areas staff working in private residential homes collect the pads once a week. In nursing homes the home is responsible for buying the pads.

Disposing of incontinence pads

Used incontinence pads cannot be disposed of with normal household waste. Homes have a duty under the Environmental Protection Act 1990 to ensure that pads are disposed of properly.

(a)

(b)

Fig. 13.8 Marsupial pants are washable; a pad is inserted into a plastic pouch and changed when wet: (a) male marsupial pants; (b) female marsupial pants.

Homes use different systems to dispose of incontinence pads. Some homes use a macerator; the pads are placed in the macerator and are reduced to a pulp and washed away into the drain. Other homes use a yellow bag system. All body waste which is to be taken away from the home and disposed of should be

Fig. 13.9 An incontinence pad held in position by specially designed pants.

collected in a yellow plastic bag. These bags are stored in special sack holders in the sluice room. The bags are either collected by the local council or by a private firm. Homes are charged for each sack of clinical waste removed. The waste is then incinerated at high temperature.

Penile sheaths

Penile sheaths look like condoms (Fig. 13.10). They are attached to the penis using either a special adhesive or a strap; the lower end has an outlet which is connected to a catheter bag. The bag is strapped to the leg. Urine drains from the penis into the catheter bag. Some men find this convenient and comfortable, whilst others do not. Penile sheaths should be removed daily. Particular care must be taken to enable the patient to maintain personal hygiene. Sheaths can cause soreness and this can lead to infection. If the patient's skin appears red or sore, carers should seek professional help.

It is important that carers listen to the patient and seek professional help if the patient finds a penile sheath uncomfortable or would prefer to use a different method to contain incontinence.

Catheters

Catheters are inserted through the urethra and into the bladder. They are held in place by a balloon which is filled with sterile

Fig. 13.10   Urinary sheath.

water. Urine is drained from the bladder by the catheter and is collected in a catheter bag. Professional staff avoid using catheters simply to contain incontinence. They are used only when no other method of controlling incontinence will be effective. People who suffer from overflow incontinence, who have failed to respond to treatment or who are too frail for surgery may have their incontinence managed by using a catheter. People who have a catheter can develop problems. These include blockage, leaking, pain and infection. If problems occur, carers should seek professional advice.

Catheter bags

Urine drains from the catheter into a catheter bag (Fig. 13.11a). There are two different types of catheter bag for night and day use. Night drainage bags are large bags. They are supported on stands which sit on the floor beside the bed. Leg bags are worn during the day (Fig. 13.11b). These are strapped to the patient's leg and hidden by either a skirt or trousers. It is important to support catheter bags by using either a stand or strapping them to the leg. Catheter bags fill with urine and can become very heavy. If the bag is not supported the weight of urine can pull the catheter and cause the neck of the bladder, where the balloon sits, to become bruised and swollen. This can cause pain and bleeding.

(a)

(b)

Fig. 13.11 (a) Catheter and drainage bag; (b) catheter and leg bag.

Emptying catheter bags

Catheter bags should be emptied every four hours. If the person is passing a lot of urine they may need to be emptied more frequently. The bag should be emptied before it is completely full to avoid pulling on the delicate tissues at the neck of the bladder.

Homes have different procedures for emptying catheters. In some homes carers wear disposable gloves to empty catheter bags. In others the carer washes her hands before and after emptying the bag. Urine should be drained into a jug which has been sterilised in the bedpan washer. The urine is then tipped down the bedpan washer and the jug resterilised.

How often should catheter bags be changed?

The Department of Health recommends that catheter bags are changed twice each week. It can be difficult for staff to keep track of when a catheter bag was last changed as one carer may change the bag before going off duty for a few days. The carer returning from days off may be unaware of this and may change the bag again. In some homes when a bag is changed the date of the change is written discreetly on the inner side of the bag with a marking pen, as well as recorded on the care plan.

Bowel care

The large bowel is known as the colon. It absorbs water and salts and the remaining waste product, faeces, is passed into the rectum. When we eat, the contents of the bowel move into the rectum. We then feel that the rectum is full and we need to open our bowels. This is known as the gastrocolic reflex. This reflex is strongest after breakfast.

Constipation

Constipation can occur if the older person does not go to the toilet when the rectum is full. The older person may, because of a loss of sensation, be unaware of the need to go to the toilet, or they may be reluctant to open their bowels. This may be because there is little privacy in the home or they feel rushed. Perhaps they have haemorrhoids and opening the bowels causes pain.

Constipation can also occur if the person's diet does not have enough fibre. Advice on a high fibre diet is given in Chapter 12. If the person is not drinking enough fluid, this can also lead to constipation. People who are not active and who do not walk about are more likely to suffer from constipation. Helping and encouraging the older person to walk will often help prevent constipation.

If the older person remains constipated despite eating a high fibre diet, drinking enough fluid and moving around, professional advice should be sought. The nurse, doctor or continence adviser will investigate the reasons for constipation and form a treatment plan. This will include checking the medication which the older person is taking. Some medication can cause constipation.

Diarrhoea

Diarrhoea is the frequent passage of loose or liquid stools. The commonest causes of diarrhoea are laxatives, antibiotics, food poisoning and faecal impaction.

Laxatives
Laxatives can be given to treat constipation, but it can be extremely difficult to calculate the dose required to enable an individual to have a normal bowel action. If the older person is eating a diet high in fibre, drinking sufficient fluids and encouraged to move around, laxatives will seldom be required.

Antibiotics
Antibiotics given to treat an infection can often cause diarrhoea. Carers who wash their hands before and after attending to each patient can reduce the number of infections older people suffer and reduce the need for antibiotics.

Food poisoning
Food poisoning can cause diarrhoea. If carers do not carefully wash their hands after attending to each patient, and do not maintain patient hygiene and carefully dispose of body fluids according to the home's policy, they can contribute to an outbreak of diarrhoea within the home.

Constipation can also lead to diarrhoea. Hard, dried faeces build up in the rectum and cannot be passed. Further faeces gather behind this and can leak around the blockage. Although it appears that the person has diarrhoea, severe constipation is the real problem.

Caring for the person with diarrhoea
If the older person develops diarrhoea, carers should seek professional help. Treatment will depend on the cause of the diarrhoea. The older person may no longer require laxatives if they are causing the problem. It may be possible for the doctor to change the antibiotic the person is taking if this is causing the diarrhoea. The person with food poisoning may require treatment if the diarrhoea is severe. The person with severe constipation will require treatment to clear the bowel.

It is important that carers encourage the patient with diarrhoea to drink plenty of fluids as extra fluid is being lost through the faeces and this must be replaced. The person who has diarrhoea may need assistance to get to the toilet in time. In some cases a commode by the bed will be required. The patient's privacy and dignity should be maintained at all times and air fresheners should be used to ensure the room does not smell, as this could embarrass the individual.

Most homes now have a policy for dealing with soiled linen – normally red plastic bags with an alginate strip. Soiled linen is placed in the red bag which is taken to the laundry where it is laundered separately from all other linen. The bag is normally placed in the washing machine and placed on sluice cycle. The alginate strip then dissolves and the bag opens. The laundry is rinsed and the bag is then disposed of. The linen is then washed normally.

Stoma care

A stoma is a piece of bowel which has been brought to the surface of the abdomen (Fig. 13.12). The stoma normally looks pink or red. The stoma takes the place of the anus and faeces pass through the stoma. The person with a stoma has no control over when the faeces will come out and must wear a bag to collect faeces (Fig. 13.13). The stoma is made from the large bowel. The large bowel absorbs water so the stool of a person with a colostomy will resemble a normal stool. The person with a colostomy uses a closed bag. When the person has passed a stool the bag is removed and replaced with a new bag.

A person who has a stoma formed from the small intestine (known as an ileostomy) will pass a liquid stool. The amount of stool will be greater and people who have ileostomies will need to drink extra fluid because of this. People who have ileostomies normally wear a drainage bag and the stool is drained into a jug.

Disposing of body waste

If the older person has a stoma there are normally two different methods of disposing of the body waste. All stoma bags come complete with a small bag with two handles. The bag is designed to hold the stoma bag and then tie up. This sealed bag is then placed in the yellow clinical waste container. In some homes faeces are tipped out of the bag and disposed of in the bedpan washer. The empty bag is then placed in a bag, sealed and placed in the yellow clinical waste bag.

If the older person has an ileostomy, the faecal fluid is normally drained into a special jug that is usually named, e.g. Mrs Jones, stomal effluent only. The fluid is disposed of in the bedpan washer. The jug is then re-sterilized for future use. This jug is kept separate from others and is never used to drain urine from catheter bags.

(a)

(b)

Fig. 13.12 (a) Normal digestive system; (b) intestines before and after a colostomy.

Summary

Enabling and helping the older person to use the toilet can prevent incontinence. Investigation and treatment can help many older people regain continence. Some older people are unable to regain continence and it is important that carers help to contain incontinence and help prevent skin problems. Older people may feel embarrassed about requiring help to use the toilet or to deal with incontinence. Great sensitivity is required and the carer's attitude

Fig. 13.13   A selection of stoma bags.

is of prime importance in helping older people accept help whilst maintaining self-esteem.

Portfolio preparation

- Identify ways in which older people living in your home are helped to maintain continence.
- Find out if the home has a continence assessment sheet and ask for a copy.
- Ask if there are patients in the home who suffer from different types of incontinence. Read their care plans and compare treatments.
- Find out how staff record details of patient's bowel actions.

- Ask what treatment is normally given for constipation.
- Gather further information from the sources listed in this chapter, to include in your portfolio.

Further reading

There are a number of books dealing with the subject of continence promotion and the management of incontinence. The books listed are suitable for carers. Carers may be able to obtain these either from the library of the college where they are studying or from the local library.

Fader, M. & Norton C. (1994) *Caring for continence.* Hawker Publications Ltd, 13 Park House, 140 Battersea Park Road, London SW11 4NB. This book has been written specially for care assistants studying at NVQ levels 2 and 3.

Castledean, C.M. & Duffin, H. (1991) *Staying Dry: Advice for Sufferers of Incontinence.* Quay Publishing, 11 Victoria Wharf, St George's Quay, Lancaster LA1 1GA. This book is aimed at people who suffer from incontinence. It is simple and easy to understand and carers will find it useful.

Norton, C. (1986) *Nursing for Continence.* Beaconsfield Publishers Ltd, 20 Chiltern Hills Road, Beaconsfield, Buckinghamshire HP9 1PL. This is a more detailed book which has been written for the trained nurse with an interest in continence care. Carers who wish to study the subject in greater depth may wish to study this book. Although it is written for trained nurses it is easy to read and a full explanation of all terms is given.

Telephone help-lines

A number of organizations and companies who supply incontinence products have a telephone service. People suffering from incontinence, carers or trained staff can telephone and ask for advice.

The Bard help-line is open from 12.30PM–4.30PM Monday to Friday. Telephone 0800 591 783.

Coloplast Service help-line is open from 9AM–7.30PM Monday to Friday. Telephone 0800 622 124.

Hollister Incare help-line is open from 9AM–5PM Monday to Friday. Telephone 0800 521 377.

The incontinence information help-line is run by a charity and offers advice and help. The lines are open from 2PM–7PM. Telephone 0191 0050.

Further information

The Alzheimer's Disease Society
158–160 Balham High Road
London SW12 9BN.
Telephone 0181 675 6557.

This society produces a booklet and a leaflet on caring for people with dementia who have continence problems. Send a large SAE, with two first class stamps.

The Continence Foundation
2 Doughty Street
London WC1N 2PH.
Tel: 0171 404 6875

The Continence Foundation produces a great deal of information on continence care, including a booklet on maintaining bowel control.

The British Colostomy Association
38–39 Eccleston Square
London SW1V 1PB.
Telephone 0171 828 5715

This charity offers information and advice to people who have colostomies, and produces a number of useful leaflets. It also provides a network of volunteers who are themselves colosto-mists. The volunteers will come and visit and provide advice and support to patients who have colostomies.

Glossary

Anaemia: A reduction in the number of red cells or the amount of haemoglobin (the substance in red blood cells which carries oxygen); causes of anaemia include poor diet and bleeding.

Alzheimer's disease: A progressive disorder of the brain. It causes total disintegration of the personality and eventually the person loses the ability to reason and to carry out the activities of daily living. There is no known cure for this terminal disease.

Angina: Lack of oxygen to the heart muscle caused by narrowing or blockage of the arteries supplying the heart with blood.

Anomia: Difficulty in finding words.

Aphasia: Inability to speak.

Arthritis: Pain, stiffness and sometimes inflammation of one or more joints.

Asthma: Narrowing of the bronchial tubes which allow air into the lungs. Caused by allergies including medication, dust and pollen. Treated with tablets and inhalers which help the bronchial tubes to relax and open, allowing air to pass freely into the lungs.

Bladder dysreflexia: *See* over-active bladder.

Cataract: The lens of the eye, which we look through in order to see clearly, becomes white, cloudy and milky in appearance. This affects the vision and can, depending on how severe it is, lead to visual problems or blindness. Treatment is surgical. The cataract is removed and usually a contact lens is inserted into the eye to replace the lens which has been removed.

Catheter (urinary): A tube which passes from the urethra to the bladder and is used to drain urine.

Cellulitis: Inflammation of tissue. This term is normally used to refer to an inflammation of the skin.

Cerebrovascular accident: A medical term for a stroke.

Colles' fracture: A fracture of the wrist.

Constipation: No bowel action for three days or more or passing very hard dry stools which may resemble rabbit droppings.

Decubitus ulcer: Medical term used for pressure sore.

Deep vein thrombosis: A clot which forms in either the deep veins of the legs or pelvis. This clot can break off and travel around the body until it becomes stuck in an artery. This is known as a pulmonary embolus. People who are immobile are at risk of developing a deep vein thrombosis.

Dementia: *See* Alzheimer's disease and multi-infarct dementia.

Diabetes: This is known as diabetes mellitus (sweet diabetes) because the urine contains sugar. This condition was first described by the ancient Greeks who diagnosed it by tasting the urine. The body is unable to use glucose (sugar) because of absence or shortage of insulin. Treatment is either by diet, so that the overweight diabetic loses weight and there is enough insulin to go round, or tablets to make the body produce more insulin, or insulin injections. Untreated diabetes leads to high levels of sugar in the blood. These high sugar levels can cause kidney damage, blindness and circulation problems.

Dysarthria: Difficulty in forming and articulating words.

Dysphasia: Difficulty in speaking or understanding words. *See* expressive dysphasia and receptive dysphasia.

Electrolytes: Balance of chemicals in the blood. These can become unbalanced because of disease, medication or poor diet.

Expressive dysphasia: General difficulty in expressing what a person wishes to say.

Fracture: A broken bone.

Gastrostomy: An opening from the stomach to the skin. This is created by a surgeon to enable nursing staff to feed people who are unable to swallow. A tube is placed into this opening and special liquid feeds are given.

Glaucoma: An eye condition which causes the pressure within the eye to become raised. There are a number of different types of glaucoma. Glaucoma can be treated medically or surgically. Untreated glaucoma can cause blindness.

Hemiplegia: Paralysis of one side of the body usually as the result of a stroke or injury to the brain.

Incontinence: The inability to 'hold on' to urine or faeces until a suitable place can be found to empty the bladder or bowel.

Intravenous infusion: This is commonly known as a 'drip'. Sterile fluid is given slowly into a vein.

Ketones: Substances which are produced within the body and removed in the urine when the body is burning fat. Seen in poorly controlled diabetics, people who have been vomiting and in starvation.

Motor neurone disease: A progressive degenerative condition. The neurones (nerve cells) degenerate leading to paralysis and eventually death. There is no known cure.

Multi-infarct dementia: Interruption of the blood supply to the brain by a small clot, causing tissue death. These small clots cause brain tissue to die and the person loses the ability to reason and function if treatment is not effective. Treatment, such as control of high blood pressure and giving a small dose of aspirin, aims to prevent clots forming in the circulation of the brain.

Nasogastric tube: A tube which goes down the nose and into the stomach. It is used to give fluids directly into the stomach when a person is unable to swallow, perhaps because of a stroke or motor neurone disease.

Osteo-arthritis: Arthritis of the hands, knees, hips and big toes.

Osteo-porosis: Thinning and weakening of the bones which makes them fracture more easily.

Overactive bladder: The bladder muscle contracts before it is completely full. The person passes small amounts of urine frequently and may find it difficult to hold on until the toilet can be reached. This can be caused by strokes or Parkinson's disease.

Overflow incontinence: Difficulty in emptying the bladder completely caused by a blockage. Constipation, Parkinson's disease and an enlarged prostate are some of the causes of overflow incontinence.

Parkinson's disease: A brain disorder caused by a reduction of a chemical, called dopamine, in the brain. It is a progressive disease and eventually the person loses the ability to carry out the activities of daily living. It causes difficulty in moving and speaking. In the early stages medication helps control symptoms.

Penile sheath: A condom-like device which fits over the penis and drains urine into a catheter bag.

Pressure sore: An area of tissue which has died because unrelieved pressure has caused the circulation to the tissue to be cut off. Pressure sores can affect skin, fat, muscle and bone, depending on the severity.

Pulmonary embolus: A clot which forms in the deep veins of the leg or pelvic veins, breaks off and travels to the heart. It can cause death by blocking a heart valve or the pulmonary artery. A smaller clot can damage lung tissue.

Receptive dysphasia: Difficulty or inability to make sense of messages received by speech.

Rheumatoid arthritis: Arthritis affecting the shoulders, wrists, fingers and toes.

Shearing forces: Damage to the capillary circulation caused by dragging or friction. The damage caused can lead to pressure sores developing.

Specific gravity: A way of checking how concentrated urine is. This enables staff to discover if a person is not having enough fluid.

Stoma: A stoma is an opening from the inside of the body to the outside. A colostomy is an opening created by a surgeon from the large bowel (colon) to the surface of the abdomen. An ileostomy is an opening from the small bowel (ileum) to the surface of the abdomen. Body waste which comes out of these stomas is collected in a bag.

Stress incontinence: A leak of urine on moving, coughing or sneezing. Caused by weakness of the muscles in the pelvic floor.

Stroke: An interruption of the blood supply to the brain caused by either bleeding or a clot. This leads to an area of tissue death and also bruising to brain tissue.

Index